THE JANUS DOCTOR

JAMES J. SCHEINER, M.D.

The names of the individuals and medications mentioned in this narrative, except for the author's,

are fictitious.

jmmmad@aol.com

ISBN: 1475107633
ISBN 13: 9781475107630

for my precious Marcy and the "four"

I would like to thank a very dear friend, Lori Tieso, a talented and courageous young woman without whom this story would never have been made known.

In Roman mythology, the god *Janus* was delegated a myriad of tasks. He was the guardian of entries, exits, and passages, was responsible for all beginnings and endings, and was the deity of the past, present, and future. He was portrayed as a human figure, but with two faces looking in opposite directions.

In modern English usage, Janus is a metaphor for simultaneous, contradictory attributes that often suggest deception. Thus, it is an appropriate term for impaired physicians who are, indeed, two-faced. The face presented toward patients and colleagues represents altruism and is moral, sincere, careful, strong, sober, and helpful. The other is the face of malevolence and dereliction. It is immoral, deceitful, careless, weak, intemperate, and neglectful.

It is a sad state of affairs, but nowadays those who must enter a hospital or clinic will surely, somewhere along the line, come face to face with a Janus doctor—and that is truly frightening.

This is the story of the Janus doctor who was me.

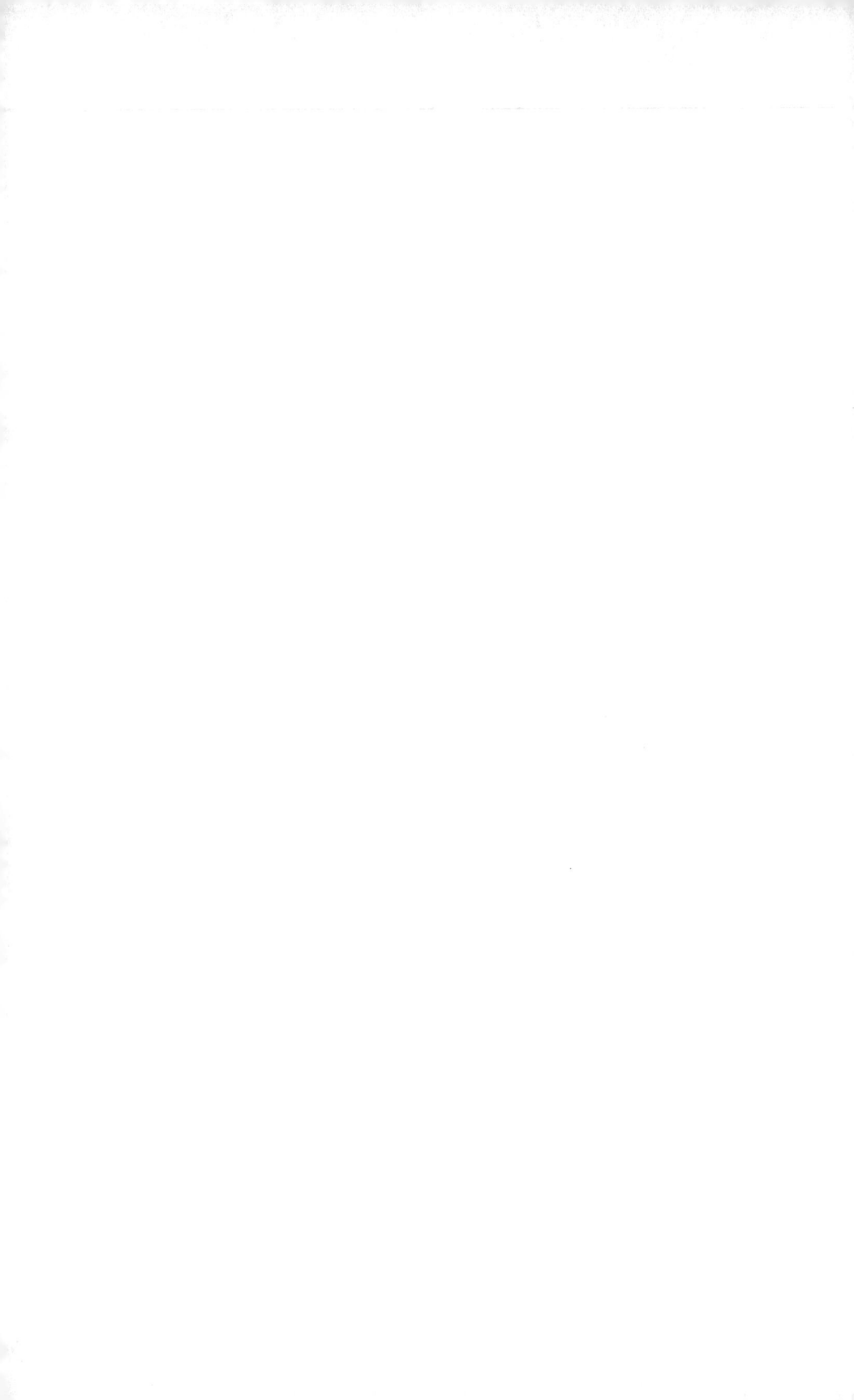

DAY OF ATONEMENT

Consumed by the crushing torment of the day's events, I found myself emotionally dead—suspended deep in the blackness of an abyss—far removed from reality. I wasn't even shamed by the brace of bullheaded, federal marshals steering and shouldering me down the slosh-covered, back steps of the now-empty courthouse. And dressed only in an oversize, brilliant-orange jumpsuit stenciled with huge, black letters that flaunted it was the "PROPERTY OF ALEXANDRIA JAIL," I wasn't even conscious of the cutting chill that had overtaken that black, starless night.

Cuffed and shackled, I could only hobble, so it took some time, for what seemed to be a small party of desperate fugitives, to get to the curbed Plymouth sedan blanketed with snow and ice. When we finally reached it, my already bowed head was emphatically pushed down even further to permit entry into the back seat. As the engine fired up, I began to tremble. I was frightened—not only because I had the devil to pay, but because I knew I faced the sinister aura of withdrawal.

Before closing my eyes in a delusive attempt to escape my impending doom, I glanced at my left wrist. The luminous face of my $15,000, platinum Breitling, now curiously coupled with a strangulating, steel cuff, showed the time to be exactly 8:20 p.m. and the date, December 21, 1980.

It had been the longest and the most god-awful day. A lifetime had passed since morning when I had sat staring straight ahead, shock-still, and anguished beside Hannah as she drove her imposing, black, 560SEL Mercedes from our Fairfax estate to the United States District Court for the Eastern District of Virginia on Washington Street in Old Town Alexandria—there, to be sentenced.

Glassy-eyed and drained, she had occasionally glanced over at me, smiling faintly: a breathing Mona Lisa. She was in a trance—half-aware and half-asleep—driving by remote. I returned her smiles being careful to avert her eyes. Instead, I looked at her hair, an undisciplined, titillating, raven mane that had recently begun to gray, and I remembered how during sex, when she was on top, it would rise and fall—untamed, rebellious, and out of control—until, sweating and moaning, she climaxed, shuddered and fell forward, exhausted. I also noted that her make-up was no longer able to hide the crow's feet she so despised, and for which she had seriously considered plastic surgery. But, more visible, even palpable, was the fact that I had emptied her of the joys of her life. I had made her age, mentally and physically, too soon.

She drove in silence. There was really nothing to say, for it had all been said and all the tears shed. And by now, she had resigned herself to the bitter fact that she would be driving back alone.

The absurdity and the pointlessness of my contemptible behavior had made it increasingly difficult to face her, not to mention the boys. I could no longer bear to tear at their hearts by making them suffer my pathetic, unpardonable shortcomings, and the evils that had led to my destruction. By existing and wallowing in nothing but self-gratification for over a decade, I had wounded and scarred them, and just about everyone else who had ever needed me or loved me. Unfortunately, I had discovered this sober truth—the destiny of a Janus doctor—way too late. And so, for the last month or so, I had remained in solitude with my misery, my self-loathing, and my rage.

We arrived at the courthouse just as the first snowflakes, like myself, had begun their descent to nothingness. With dread and near panic, I soon found myself in Courtroom 2, an enormous, glaringly lighted, domed chamber swarming with both those who upheld the law and those who dared laugh in its face. Before we could even sit down, the bailiff thundered: "Docket number 81 – 00220 – A: United States of America v. James J. Scheiner, M.D." The sudden silence and the fact that everyone's eyes were fixed on me were unnerving. My lawyer, appearing out of nowhere, took my arm and prodded me to a small lectern that served as the dock. It had been placed in the center of the room facing the judge's remote, lofty throne, and surrounded on all sides by time-worn benches jammed with villains and scoundrels of every age, breed, and genre awaiting the inevitable. Here, seated quietly, as if in church, were the dregs of society, and each and every one was now my peer.

With my heart leaping in my mouth and in a cold sweat, I gripped the lectern and forced myself to look up. It was over in no time. After a brief but decisive chastisement that wound up with, "To me, there is nothing as repugnant than those who, entrusted with the lives of their fellow men, corrupt that privilege. Nothing." With unconcealed contempt, the judge sentenced me to a term of seven years in a federal penitentiary, three years of supervised probation, and a $30,000 fine. But, perhaps convinced of my undisguised contrition and humility, he suspended six years of the prison term.

Somehow I managed to turn around to face Hannah. As she stood up—slowly and alone—I saw her pallid, tear-stained face. She was trembling. I thought she might collapse. We stared at each other for a moment, and then she haltingly raised an arm in farewell, smiled listlessly, shook her head, turned around, and walked out.

Suddenly, everything was blurred and muted. I was about to black out when someone grabbed my wrists, cuffed them behind my back, and then led me to a small jail cell somewhere in the bowels of that courthouse—there, to begin a life of pain and humiliation. Just before leaving the courtroom, however, I'd noticed several suited spectators in the rear gleefully giving each other "high-fives." One of them was the FDA agent whose unrelenting investigation of my criminal transgressions had led to this day.

It was strange, paradoxical, but immediately upon being locked up and set apart from everything and everyone, I felt relieved. And, for the first time I could ever recall, free! Time and life seemed to be of no concern. It was as if, all of a sudden, I had been purged of every emotion, sensation, hope, and dream. I had literally ceased to be.

Drained, I managed to clamber up a naked, corrugated, metal ledge about four feet off the floor, the only fixture in that cage apart from a seatless, steel commode, and instantly fall asleep. I'm not sure how long I slept, but I awoke with a start and, for a moment, confused as to where I was. I struggled off that excuse for a bed, my entire body stiff and throbbing, and proceeded to examine my Spartan courthouse basement surroundings.

I was inside one of a line of three cells that faced a narrow hallway encased on either end by heavy steel doors fitted at eye level with small, green-tinted, chicken-wired windows. In the cobwebbed corners above the doors, TV monitors silently rotated. The wall of the hallway contained two small, heavily barred windows through which the amber after-glow of the day diffused. The softened, almost-dreamy rays illuminated the restless dust particles suspended in the dry, stagnant air that reeked of commercial disinfectant. Aside from the occasional clank of a distant radiator, and the ominous ticking of a clock somewhere, there was silence. I was alone, and my ephemeral feelings of relief turned to fear.

Just as I completed my surveillance, the quiet was abruptly disturbed by the arrival of two, sphinx-like, Stetson hatted Neanderthals.

Obsessed by my plight, I was oblivious to the movement of the car as it forged its way through the muddied slush, fast-accumulating on the narrow, cobbled streets. Before it had gone any distance, however, I was jolted out of my trance, as well as my seat, when it skidded on a patch of ice and crashed into the left, rear fender of a black XJ12 sedan.

After backing off the Jaguar's crumpled fender with the shattered, useless, tail light, the Neanderthal behind the wheel, without so much as a blink, continued on. As he surged into the frenzied currents of traffic on I-95 South, I was suddenly besieged by the simultaneous agony of savage hunger and a merciless bladder. I hadn't eaten, drunk, or peed all day. And then, my hopelessly incorrigible ulcer—a legacy of years of stress and drugs—erupted into flame. I could see in my mind's eye the crimson, swollen lining of my stomach embracing a massive crater spewing acid like an erupting volcano.

At odds with each other, the paroxysms of the varied pains became insufferable. I became soaked with sweat, and my face, twisted and teary. I needed food, water, medicine, and, more than anything, a bathroom; basic needs I had once secured with no real effort or thought. I realized with dread that I was no longer in a position to assuage my own body's needs and no longer in a position to request or demand them. For so many years, as an arrogant, presumptuous surgeon with money to burn, I knew I could have whatever I wanted. I now was reduced to nothing less than a trapped creature—helpless and dependent.

I leaned forward to ask where and when we would reach our destination. My body's festering anguish made it difficult and painful to speak. My throat was on fire. The now nonstop stream of acid had made its way all the way up to my mouth. I yelled as loud as I could over the deafening blast of country-western the two cowboys upfront had been listening to ever since we left Alexandria. Receiving no answer, I at first thought the music had drowned out my raucous voice. But after the "six-in-a-row" series of vocals ended for a commercial break, I heard a single word—"Petersburg."

"When?"

"Two hours. Now shut the fuck up!"

And then I lost it. I became a savage—foaming at the mouth, wild-eyed. I was in a rage and screamed at the top of my voice: "Fuck you, too, you sons of bitches." Too late, I realized my mistake. The cowboy in the passenger's seat turned around, reached over, and slapped me with a hand as big as a catcher's mitt hard across the face. "The next time you open your fuckin' trap," he warned, "I'll break your jaw . . . DOCTOR!" As I sat back and swallowed a mouthful of blood, I knew that my outburst was an omen. The dreaded, pitiless chaos of withdrawal was about to burst forth.

Shortly past midnight, the Plymouth turned onto an unmarked road which, after about a half mile, dead ended at a massive, barred gate, curtaining a dark and threatening tunnel. Extending for an unseeable span from each side of the gate was a towering, chain-link fence capped with ugly, razor-sharp, accordion wire. Every few seconds the radiant flash of a Klieg light, emanating high above the center of this sinister compound, cleaved the darkness. Its brilliance exposed dimly lit watchtowers at each corner and caused the ugly wire to sparkle.

The car again skidded, missing the gate by a hair. Then it shuddered and died, creating a silence, heavy with impending menace. The Neanderthal on the passenger side got out, violently jerked open my door, reached in, yanked me out, and pushed me to the gate, where he hammered at a Klaxon-like buzzer until a lethargic, yawning guard dragged himself out of the tunnel. They exchanged papers, without a word. Then my travel companions drove off in their government car with the huge dent in the right front fender and a smashed, darkened headlight. The already ungodly angst of this day now became even further heightened by the awful, oppressive darkness, desolation, and silence. Standing there in the bitter cold, I could feel what was left of my life energy melt away. I had truly arrived at hell's gate.

A migraine hammered savagely in concert with my bladder behind my eyes as I waited, shivering, in the gloom of the Gothic tunnel leading into the prison. As I stood, teetering and drooping, my mind began to drift. From its deepest, most-secret recesses, it began to surrender forgotten memories of another prison long ago.

ROOTS

Golda Bensinger, a somewhat seductive, auburn-haired Pole, was born with all the charms of a scorpion. In 1926, at the age of 16, she, along with her parents and sisters—Getel and Ruth—sailed in steerage to America. Following their run through at the Federal Immigration Station on Ellis Island, they continued by train to Cleveland to join the thousands of other Polish "refujews" who had been swarming there since the turn of the century. Most, like the Bensingers, had come with nothing, except the memories of a joyless existence and the expectation of finding, as they had been led to believe, streets paved with gold, but which, they soon discovered, were nothing but boulevards of blighted dreams.

I once asked her, "Ma, how come we have nothing in our house from Poland? Didn't you bring anything with you when you came here?"

"What do you mean, nothing?!" she snapped, knowing full well what I meant.

"You know, like pictures or souvenirs."

"I don't know. Maybe, everything got lost. Maybe, on the ship or at the Ellis Island." Then, after a moment, she blinked wildly, smiled sadly, and murmured, "Actually, Yosele, we brought nothing so we would be able to soon forget the terrible life we were leaving. But, even so, there are things one never forgets."

I could see her tears as she hurried out of the room and, young as I was, knew better than to ask, "What things?"

❧

The Bensingers settled in a tenement flat on Cleveland's East 130th and Kinsman, in the heart of a square mile of neglect and filth that was never free of impenetrable herds of brassy, boorish humanity. In fact, it was not unlike the groveling, contemptuous ghetto they had just left behind in Warsaw. Regardless of her punishing circumstances, however, Golda was a proud woman. Throughout her childhood, her parents and teachers had literally drilled into her mind that she was one of the chosen people, an Orthodox Jew, and that being so was spiritually, morally, and racially superior to all other members of the human race.

To help her family make ends meet, Golda found work as a seamstress in a sweatshop that made shirtwaists. When she was 19, one of her fellow wage slaves introduced her to Morris Scheiner, a tall, handsome, curly haired, charismatic young baker who, contrary to his peers, had a perfect Roman nose and cared nothing of religion. Golda found him to be a welcome relief from the shabby, smelly, jobless, repulsive, chauvinistic, pious, little greenhorns her father, a brushfaced, dandruff-laden, seedy-looking, do-nothing rabbi would have her marry.

Nathan, though intelligent, for some reason lacked purpose. Shallow and irresolute, he was content to remain on the sidelines of life looking in. He had no friends or even family ties, and, other than the Cleveland Indians and liquor, he had no interests, not even in his livelihood. It was Nathan's phlegmatic, antithetical temperament that captured Golda's fancy. He was, apparently, just what she had been looking for in a partner: a beast of burden she could lead by the nose, and in so doing, have it all her own way. Her agenda was that he would work and she would keep him happy in bed until such time enough money had been socked away to realize her objective. She wanted a business of her own—a bakery.

They were married by a Justice of the Peace on May 6, 1933, and set up housekeeping in a cold-water dump in a tenement at the corner of East 105th and Euclid Avenue. Mantled with decades of guano, the tenement, like all the others in that urban *shtetl* of a neighborhood, was a six-story cube of architectural ennui corrupted by window ledges crammed with a jumble of precariously balanced, potted, grieving plants and decaying foodstuffs packed in boxes, jars, bottles, and bags. A rusting fire escape zigzagged down one wall, interrupting a maze of clotheslines, always heavy with wash, strung between adjoining cubes. Inside, all was stink, gloom, and dissonance—garbage, urine, slamming doors, shouts, curses, screams, weeping, and shadows.

Their flat on the top floor was nothing more than a box divided by nearly transparent walls into four smaller boxes: a kitchen, a bedroom, a parlor, and a bathroom. The kitchen, with its two-burner stove, was the only room that was, in some measure, warm during the winters. It was there, my older sister, Regina, born December, 1934, and I, a year and a half younger, slept on verminous mattresses. There were no closets or chests of drawers, so our clothes sprawled in careless piles on the floor or dangled from scattered doorknobs.

Although we were a two-income family, we remained starkly poor by design, since mother was busy saving according to her Plan "A." Both she and my father must have been putting in long hours since, until we moved away from there in 1944, I scarcely ever saw them. We did nothing together. Outings, vacations, and restaurants were unheard of, as were family dinners, other than on those rare occasions when my mother would prepare, on Friday night, Sabbath eve, a meal of bland, boiled chicken, the slimy, sticky, scaly feet of which, for some reason, always found their way onto my plate.

It was Regina, my older sister, who, while still a toddler, instinctively assumed the role of mother and kept me from becoming a feral beast. Sensible and wise beyond her years, she afforded me and, later, the four other children in our family, the only security we ever knew as children. She prepared our simple meals—sandwiches, hot dogs and beans, or just beans—and kept our baby bottles filled with milk. Somehow, too, she got the dimes we needed to go to the movies on Saturdays. We parked ourselves there most of the day, watching the movies two, sometimes three times over, while munching the sandwiches we had snuck in (since there was never extra money for popcorn or soda pop).

And it was Regina who got me up at daybreak, one day every August, to take me to the annual milkman's picnic at the Euclid Beach Amusement Park on Lake Shore Boulevard where all the rides, that day, were free. To this day, I still wonder how she knew how to get there, since three trolleys were needed. When she first took me, she was only six.

Just before my fourth birthday, my mother, as a matter of course and custom, enrolled me in a *heder*, a parochial school for Jewish boys. It wasn't much of a school—simply one, poorly furnished, cramped classroom in the basement of an abandoned fish market. The once white, stuccoed plaster walls were a snarl of fissures, stains, and smudges. Even during the summer, it was cold and damp and never free of the pervasive stink of long-dead fish.

My first teacher, Rabbi Gross, a brooding, penniless, chain-smoking, religious zealot who had recently escaped the sorry life of a *shtetl* just outside Bialystok near the Russian border, was a tragic specimen of a man. Although only 30 or so, a bout of childhood tuberculosis had left him with a grotesque hump on his back and a stunted, shriveled body. His magnificent carrot-colored beard that set off the bluest, saddest eyes I had ever seen, couldn't quite conceal a butchered attempt to correct a harelip. Although he had the conviction, he had absolutely no concept as to how to teach children. I and a handful of classmates, for three hours five afternoons a week, just slouched around a scarred, oak table, in dim light, suppressing yawns while trying to make some sense of the sacred words written by ancient Hebraic scholars in fusty moldering Talmuds and Pentateuchs.

I hated being there. It was tedious and exasperating, made even more so by the realization that while I was being closeted every day after public school in some sort of nether world, the Christian kids were outside playing, eating ice cream and Mars bars, and otherwise having fun. The *heder* was a torment for me that lasted the better part of 12 years.

Other than on Yom Kippur, the holiest Jewish holiday, my parents never set foot in a synagogue. We, of course, had Jewish neighbors, but all of them remained sequestered in their own lives. There was no sense of community or solidarity. It was a reclusive, obscure, seemingly xenophobic existence, without encouragement or inspiration from anyone. As a result, the entire time I spent at the *heder* was meaningless, wasted. The concept and need of faith eluded me. In the long run, my religious training there did more harm than good, because it only really taught me racism.

For every one of my rabbis teaching the fundamental agenda of Judaism— be merciful, love your fellow Jew, and walk without arrogance—seemed not to be enough. They felt they had to do more, and by their zeal in expressing and flaunting their faith, they crossed into the world of fanaticism and, in so doing, corrupted that basic agenda.

From the start, they proclaimed, in no uncertain terms, that we were the "chosen," since God had seen fit to reveal himself only to the Jews. This personal consecration implied that Jews were spiritually, morally, and racially superior to any other national, ethnic, or religious group on this planet. Indisputable proof of this was shown to us again and again from one end of the Bible to the other and throughout the writings of the ancient Hebrew sages until these "truths" were etched indelibly in our minds and taken for granted.

I'm sure those rabbis, in their passionate enthusiasm to serve God, meant no harm. By overvaluing the notion of the chosen, they perceived themselves to be the elect of God. In truth, though, their approach was a megalomaniacal search for omnipotence in order to conceal their weaknesses and insecurities. Because they ignored the fundamental values of Judaism—justice, mercy, and love—they ended up displaying only weakness in their belief, and, tragically, sowing the seeds of a cold, heartless attitude towards others. By refusing to acknowledge anyone outside of the chosen, and by ridiculing, shunning, or holding these outsiders in contempt, they certainly, but perhaps unknowingly, caused a great deal of emotional hurt and harm to themselves, to say nothing of their students.

I may have hated *heder* for all its oppressiveness, but at least I was accepted by the other students as a peer, which made being there somewhat tolerable. I shudder with loathing, however, at my early days in public school. From the very first day of kindergarten at Miles Standish Elementary School, I was an object of pitiless ridicule and snickering. It wasn't my fault, inasmuch as we usually spoke Yiddish at home and at the *heder*, and my exposure to English-speaking children was so inconsequential that I could barely speak or understand English. And it wasn't my fault that I looked and dressed differently from the other kids. I had to wear a *yarmulke*, and, instead of creased trousers and brightly colored shirts, I wore homely, wool knickers and cheap, white, long sleeved shirts—more often than not soiled and wrinkled. Tassels, known as *tzitzit,* sewn onto the four corners of my undershirt emerged conspicuously from my shirt, dancing and swinging to and fro, in concert with my dangling sidelocks.

Never having been taught why or how to use a toothbrush, my mouth was a perpetual scene of departed and disconnected teeth, corruption, and foul breath. Bathing and a regular change of clean underwear were, likewise, not part of my daily routine. This proved to be quite embarrassing for me and a source of head-shaking and smirks when I changed into shorts for phys-ed class. It also, of course, explained why no one had any desire to sit near me in class.

Another source of mockery was my midmorning snack. Other kids' trendy little lunch boxes contained Oreos, Twinkies, and milk or juice; my brown bag contained a glass baby bottle of milk, complete with a huge red nipple. Looking back, it's no wonder I was a laughingstock and fair game for the cruel propensities of my classmates. I always wondered, however, why the teacher never sent a note home advising my mother that maybe I was a bit old to be sucking on a bottle.

The first day of the first grade went by without incident, and as I walked home, I was filled with the hope that the crushing shame and humiliation I had suffered during kindergarten was, forever, behind me. Lamentably, it was not.

On the second day as I was getting ready to sit at my desk after morning recess, I noticed a new student seated at the desk directly in front of mine: a little girl who the teacher, Ms. Clark, introduced as Samantha Washington. I remember being somewhat muddled, since I had never before been that close to a black person. I couldn't take my eyes off the blackness of her slender neck and of her little, protruding ears, pierced with tiny pink pearl earrings. I had never before seen or even imagined such a curious head of nappy hair with its paired pigtails, all fancied up with tiny, pink and white bows that matched her homemade, striped, gingham dress.

I could hardly wait to go home for lunch so I could broadcast the news of the "colored" girl Ms. Clark had sat right in front of me. By the time I was seated in the kitchen and had begun to describe this wonder to my mother and Regina, my excitement had reached a feverish pitch. Within seconds, though, it was completely replaced by dismay and fright. Upon hearing of Samantha, my mother began to shiver so violently that the butter dish in her hand dropped to the floor. As she bent down to pick up the fragments, I watched, as her face flushed with anger, and then, like a chameleon, quickly faded into a haggard, ashen mask of fear and rage. When she was finished cleaning the floor, she began to storm all over the house; one moment, clasping her hands in her apron, the next, pressing a hand against her forehead, and all the while, fuming, sputtering, and shouting, "*A shvartze! Oi vai! Oi vai! Gott in himmel! Es ist geferlech! A shvartze!*"

Unable to comprehend her indignation, I softly asked, "Ma, why are you so mad?"

"Mad? I'm more than mad! I'm crazy mad!" she screamed.

As Regina and I pouted our lips and shrugged, she went on to say, "For ten years, I've worked and worked and saved and saved so we could leave behind those slums with their low-life Jews and *shvartze vilde khayem* (black wild animals). It's enough we have to live with the *goyim*, but *shvartzes*? *Oi vai*! Now you listen to me! You're not going back to that *meshugana* school 'til I talk to the teacher!"

All I could do was shake my head, confused and scared.

The following morning, still angry, she dragged me, embarrassed as hell, into a classroom filled with ogled eyes, dissonant giggles, small voices, closing books, and rustling papers. After a brief but heated "chat" with Ms. Clark, I found myself seated at a desk practically in the cloakroom at the rear of the classroom, my eyes filled with tears and humiliation, and my mind racked with pangs of suspicion and dread as to how and why such a tiny, spidery, bowlegged, innocent child could provoke such turmoil, and turn my mother into the very thing *she* feared—*a vilde khaye.*

BAPTISM

A prison guard kicked me. Shaken back to reality, I stared at him in disbelief. He stared back—his black eyes oblivious to my hurt. He was a scrawny, prissy caricature of a man, with a ferret's face. Right off, I could tell he fancied himself superior and self-important, but in fact he was totally devoid of dignity— typical of prison guards in general, I later found. Once we had stared each other down, he jerked his head and snarled with a lisp, "Leth go!"

He led the way out of the tunnel, across an open quadrangle, and up the steps of an ancient, fortress-like, building erratically punctuated with forbidding, barred windows into which, still in shackles, I stumbled in, still half asleep. Inside, the silence was broken from time to time by the irritating staccato of ancient radiators whose heat was flagrantly oppressive. The air was laden with commercial disinfectant—a smell I would later always associate with prison.

The ferret rudely prodded me up several flights of stairs, decisively polished and waxed as only those who have nothing but time on their hands could accomplish. We exited at the fourth floor where he unlocked the door of a small, windowless room and switched on the light. An instant Polaroid Land Camera and fingerprinting paraphernalia sat on a table, directly beneath a single, exposed, blinding light bulb. He unlocked my handcuffs, and after scrutinizing my Breitling, gently and conscientiously depressed my thumbs and each of my fingers into an ink pad, then carefully rolled them onto the designated spaces of an FBI fingerprint identification card. That done, he instructed me to hold a white, plastic card on which the numerals

1-0-2-4-3-8 had been fastened with paper clips across the front of my chest. "Memorize that number forthwith," he ordered, "because that's what you are now."

I was now fully alert. My psyche was on edge—racing—and my emotions—volatile. Helpless, frustrated, and trapped, I was overcome with shame and guilt, along with pain, hunger, and the still-urgent need to pee. And I felt my habit coming on —not yet chaotic—but an itch, staring me right in the face. Under the circumstances, I knew it was futile to ask for food or the whereabouts of a bathroom. Defeated, I just endured as the ferret put the cuffs back on and then practically shoved me all the way back down the stairs to the subterranean bowels of my new home.

We entered a narrow, far-reaching cosmos of tunnels, dimly lit by a line of bulbs held captive in metal cages. The gray-colored walls and ceilings were all but concealed by a cramped, legion of sweating, peeling, leaking, rusting pipes. It was silent, except for the rhythmic cadence of water trickling onto the concrete floor and one faint, lonesome, melancholy wail of a train, somewhere in another world. After walking for what seemed a mile, we entered a vast, cavernous chamber filled with shelves and racks overburdened with recycled military surplus uniforms. Emblazoned on every bit of exposed wall, floor, and ceiling were repulsive, lewd graffiti drawn and inscribed by generations of uncouth, crass convicts.

An old, black dwarf slouched in a creaking wheeled chair behind a small ravaged desk smoking the remnant of a reefer. He was filthy, foul-smelling, and so ugly, deformed, and repugnant I couldn't stop looking at him. He was potbellied, snaggle-toothed, and hump-backed. His enormous head was further aggrandized by a pure white "Afro." His eyes—small, intense, and bloodshot—were set close together, virtually contiguous with the bridge of a bulbous, furrowed nose.

Obviously piqued by the intrusion, the dwarf looked up, squinted, tilted his huge head, and with difficulty rose out of his chair and wordlessly proceeded to take his time gathering the requisite apparel for the new con. When he finished his task, he raised his arms and handed me a pile of olive-drab clothes with his stunted, spade-like hands with the letters H-A-T-E and L-O-V-E tattooed on the knuckles.

Trembling from revulsion, I realized I was neither more nor less than this primeval Lilliputian. Then my stomach, mercifully forgotten while all this was going on, suddenly ignited and began to flame, as did my bladder. I was sick and needed to vomit and desperately to pee.

The ferret removed my handcuffs and shackles and ordered me to strip. I undressed, dispirited and unnerved, while he watched—his tight, thin lips arced into a sardonic smirk.

Reaching into the back pocket of his perfectly fitting, sharply creased trousers, he took out a surgical glove, then deliberately fitted it on his right hand. As I stood naked and vulnerable, desperately trying not to appear unnerved, he began his painstaking examination: deliberately mussing my hair, searching the inner recesses of my armpits, thoroughly inspecting the inside of my mouth and ears. He then turned his attention to my genitalia, taking a long, hard look at my spiritless penis and gently kneading my balls.

I shuddered as I saw him once again reach into his back pocket and take out a well-crimped tube of KY Jelly. The clear, viscous lubricant made a sudden and prolonged fart-like blast as he squeezed out a generous amount onto the middle finger of his gloved hand. The dwarf—who had been gawking at all of this—was startled by the dissonance and roared in delight. This time, with an undisguised smile, the ferret motioned me to bend over, and to "spread 'em, boy!" Upon assuming this awkward and vulnerable posture, he swiftly and with a vengeance forced a trained finger up through the spastic, unyielding sphincter of my rectum, probing and reaming mercilessly. "Now thand up," he ordered, "spread your legs apart . . . farther! . . . hold your arms out . . . higher!" Satisfied with my pose, he proceeded to prance around spraying me with something that scorched my skin like the flame of a welding torch. He then patted my butt and said, "You can get 'drethed' now." By now, there was no mistaking his sexual slant.

Slowly and painfully, I stood up. By clenching my fists, biting my lips, and shutting my tearing eyes tightly, I attempted to blot out— as if it were possible—this indignity. I was exhausted, my breathing labored, and I felt depleted of lifeblood. I began to mutter over and over, "God, what the fuck have I done? What have I done to deserve this shit?" I don't know why I was asking God that question. I knew perfectly well what I had done, and that I deserved all that was coming to me, and probably more.

I knew I had no choice but to accept the reality of my plight. There were no options, and there was no escape. My punishment was immutable. I had to yield and submit to this unspeakable demotion, and to the discipline, manipulation, and ideology of those in control. I had to take my "medicine," atone for my sins, and pay my debt.

Composing myself as best I could, I slipped into the set of mismatched, ill-fitting fatigues—*sans* belt—that the dwarf had selected for me, and sadly gave up my Docksiders for a pair of throwaway canvas slip-ons. My clothes, wallet, a few coins, and the treasured Breitling—emblem of my former life as a "successful" surgeon—were then tagged and sealed in a large, brown, paper bag. The dwarf was clearly in awe of the watch, and had I not been staring at him, I'm sure he would have palmed it. Nevertheless, I somehow knew I'd never see it again.

As the dwarf carried off my personal effects a scruffy, aproned con deferentially entered the chamber, and with trembling hands set a tray of food on the desk. The ferret smiled and murmured, "Enjoy." When I saw what was on that warped, discolored, plastic tray, I was revolted: a massive chunk of spoiled, gray, disgustingly greasy and gristly meat crowning a mound of macerated cabbage, a single slice of stale white bread, and a paper cup half filled with sickly sweet strawberry Kool-Aid. Everything was cold except the drink which was lukewarm. There was no napkin, and the only utensil was a small, white, plastic spoon.

I knew I had to put something in my empty stomach to dilute and absorb the acid that was angering and scalding my ulcer. So, standing beside the desk, holding up my trousers with my left hand, and trying not to look at the dwarf, I managed to down that odious garbage.

Realizing the futility of requesting a napkin, I wiped my greasy mouth on my sleeve. The pain in my stomach had lessened, but I knew all too well that another demon was lurking—withdrawal. No longer an "itch," the craving was fast approaching a ravenous lust verging on the brink of an explosion. I was becoming irritable and hot. Sweat began to pour and I could feel my pulse racing. I had trouble focusing my tearing eyes and difficulty breathing. Every muscle in my body was aching and trembling.

After the ferret replaced my cuffs and shackles and guided me back through the remote, fetid bowels of the prison to the staircase, the long, drawn-out, violent yawns began: the tocsin giving warning that very soon the satanic symptoms of withdrawal would become unbridled—rampant and vicious.

On the sixth floor landing we passed through a barred, well-guarded antechamber, and entered a long, narrow corridor lined on both sides with darkened, silent cells. We walked to the end, stopping in front of an impregnable, remotely controlled, steel door. While waiting for it to open, I stood there, head bowed, gazing unblinkingly at the concrete floor with my hands still gripping my empty pockets in order to keep my pants up. A clock was ticking above the door; it read 3:20 a.m.

As the door slowly opened, I saw an ever-expanding view of bedlam. I recoiled, attempting to back away, but the ferret pushed me in, and the door slammed shut with an explosive, jolting, reverberating crash: a haunting, irrevocable exclamation point. I immediately searched for the toilet.

A BORN LOSER

During the entire time I lived at home, my father never made any effort to bond with me as a son. In fact, he only took me on an outing with him on one occasion.

It was during the spring of 1943 and my father had just been called to active duty. Not being much of a flag waver, he managed to get out of it by means of a scheme that I came to understand only years later, while a freshman in medical school. What I discovered then only confirmed what I had always known. He had been not only a drunk, but a coward and a fool.

I remembered it as being a comfortable spring morning. I was alone on the kitchen floor eating, as usual, an uninspiring breakfast of dry Corn Flakes directly out of the box. I frequently ate on the floor since the table teetered so badly, either because it was so lopsided, or the floor so uneven, or both. It was almost impossible to eat on it using two hands since you had to steady it with one hand or an elbow. Funny, no one ever thought to fix it, nor was anyone ever concerned that I took my meals hunkered down on the floor. In any event, my father walked in.

"Let's go, Yosele," he blurted out, "We're going to the park."

I was beside myself with delight but also mystified. He had never taken me anywhere before. Why now?

We rode three streetcars for over an hour and a half, during which he slept as if dead. He snored with a stink of stale whiskey, his clothes smelled, and he was badly in need of a bath, a shave, and a haircut.

The conductor had to wake him at the end of the line, and, finally, after we walked three or four blocks, we arrived at the doctor's office.

At that moment, I realized my father's promise of the park had been a pretense. He wanted to hide this doctor's visit from my mother. But why? Was I sick? Were they going to cut me open? I began trembling with fright. We sat there for what must have been at least two hours before a tall, withered woman with horribly bowed legs wearing a spotless nurse's uniform led us into an examining room. She sat me on a stool in a corner and handed me a lollipop.

I then sat, relieved but bewildered, as the doctor proceeded to examine my father's penis. After some treatments that seemed to cause my father agonizing pain, and which I was unable to watch, he took me to a drugstore where he handed in a prescription. While we waited for it, he bought me a chocolate ice cream sundae, and warned me never to tell my mother where we had gone because, "she'd be scared and, besides, I'm well now."

Sixteen years later, at about two o'clock in the morning, I was looking through the lens of a microscope in the microbiology lab at the University of Cincinnati College of Medicine studying the characteristic morphology of *Neisseria gonorrhoeae* when that day suddenly flashed across my mind, and it dawned on me that my father had screwed a diseased whore for the sole purpose of contracting gonorrhea so he could stay out of the army.

My father's life proved meaningless. He failed as a human being, failed even more as a father. Why this was so, and why he was an alcoholic, I will never know. In later years, when most of his brain cells had been dissolved by a tankerload of J.T.S. Brown whiskey, he became permanently lethargic, confused, and amnesic. I last saw him in a seedy, Jewish nursing home when he was 60 or so years old. He had absolutely no clue as to who I was. But then, he never did.

THE TOILET

As the massive, steel, bulkhead crashed shut behind me, splitting my eardrums and further wracking my nerves, my nose alerted me: it had to be a toilet. Bent over and just about overcome with paroxysms of racking cramps, I rushed into the room where the noxious stench was brewing, then gingerly made my way across a mostly wet floor littered with fragments of filthy toilet paper, wadded-up paper towels, hairs of various color and curl, a used-up, crimped tube of Pepsodent, and assorted cigarette wrappers, to the far wall where, at last, I saw three, doorless, toilet stalls.

An enormous, black "barge" was wedged into the stall nearest the showers. He raised his head up from his comic book, glared at me and bellowed, "What the fuck yo lookin at muthafucka? Git yo white ass away, honky shit."

I rushed into one of the empty stalls, wiped the tainted seat with a moist paper towel, and was, at long last, able to relieve myself.

As I stood up, concerned over the deplorable corruption that had just left my body, I sensed something watching me. Then, as it moved, I saw it. Directly in front of me, not three feet away, was the largest, most-repulsive looking insect I had ever seen. It was brownish-orange and heavy with slime. Its "feelers" furiously waved to and fro. We stared at each other for a while and then the creature slowly and fearlessly sauntered into the black gap between the side of the toilet stall and the wall.

After washing my hands, I flung the paper towel into a large, dented wastebasket chained to the wall under a sink. It was piled high with bathroom debris spilling over onto the floor, reminding me of the wastebasket in the mimeograph room back in the zoo building, so many years ago. Before leaving, I glanced into the mirror above the sink. It was cracked and fissured into lace-like patterns in so many spots that I had to weave and bob in order to see the various parts of my face. And when I managed to reassemble the fragmented images, I turned away in disgust.

A BIGOTED GONIF

On my ninth birthday which, like all the others, went virtually unnoticed, my Aunt Getel and her two daughters moved into our flat, specifically into the shadowy parlor where my two younger sisters—Mollie and Jennie—slept. To make room for Getel's rollaway bed and two more mattresses, the heavy chesterfield had been pushed over to one wall and the armchair, ottoman, and coffee table piled precariously on top of it.

Aunt Getel, who they say had been a comely, enchanting child, was cursed with von Recklinghausen's disease. Shortly after her fourth birthday, her skin became marred by a plethora of coffee colored splotches which, thankfully, spared her face and which wouldn't have been all that bad if, coincident with her first menstrual period, hundreds of slow-growing tumors hadn't begun to ravage her body. This time, her face was not spared. Disastrously, there was no cure, let alone treatment, for this obscene affliction.

When she was 38 years old, two crushing events took place in her life: her husband, Nicholas, a schizophrenic with uncontrollable seizures, was committed to the State Hospital for the Insane, and one of her tumors morphed into a cancer. When told she had only a few months to live, she started drinking.

Within a few days of her moving in with us, her older daughter, Elaine, who was around 13 at the time, ran away. Many years later, I learned she became a prostitute, married a black man, robbed stores, and did some jail time. Her four-year-old sister, Esther, however, spent her days with us running around like a savage beast in a filthy pair of panties, whimpering and screaming gobbledygook. Aunt Getel, seemingly too ill or drunk to control her or maybe just not giving a damn, only screamed in reply.

⁊

Before Getel and Esther arrived, life had been a dragged-out malaise. When they moved in, it became pandemonium. And so, one morning when my mother had a rare moment of beneficence or, perhaps, a need to get out of that bedlam, I was more than thankful when she asked me if I wanted to walk with her to the store. She had never asked me to go shopping with her before but had, on occasion, taken Regina. At the time, however, all three of my sisters and Esther were indisposed with chicken pox and supposedly, according to the red sign posted on the door of our flat, in quarantine.

Woolworth's five-and-ten-cent store was a vast emporium with acres of tables overflowing with a breathtaking assortment of household wares and clothing being eyed, pawed, fondled, and fought over by a surging, irrational rabble of boisterous refugees. There was a sale going on.

Once we elbowed our way inside, mother smiled inexplicably and insisted with a gentle push that I, "Go! Look around! I'll find you when I'm done." Terrified of becoming lost within that retail jungle, I made sure she was never out of my sight. Occasionally, I would chance upon her furtively glancing about like an animal in the wild trying to catch a scent, and then her impetuous fingers would snatch something off a table and thrust it into the enormous, black patent-leather pocketbook strapped around her neck. After about an hour, as I stood tiptoed, mesmerized by a display of provocative Erector sets, watching their miniaturized beams, gears, cog wheels, and motorized cables revolving wondrously around, I witnessed her "appropriate" the last item—a small red object.

Halfway home, I found out what it was. Without a word, she took my hand and placed a small, blood-red Swiss Army knife in my palm. It contained two blades, a miniature saw, scissors, and a screwdriver. It was smooth, heavy, and solid, and it felt right in my hand although my fingers were almost too small to go around it. Intoxicated, I stopped dead in my tracks. I have never forgotten that moment, because it was one of the few times in my childhood that I ever really smiled and felt love for my mother. I skipped and hopped and whistled the rest of the way home.

Knife in hand, I scampered up the six flights of stairs and flung open the kitchen door with such force that the doorknob impaled itself in the wall. Aunt Getel, wearing only a slip, was slumped, dead-drunk, over the wobbly kitchen table. An empty whiskey bottle and a water glass lay, precariously, on their sides near its edge. Under the table, Regina and Mollie, their faces red and blistered, sat eating Rice Krispies out of the box and giggling at Esther who was peeing on the floor. The odor of stale alcohol and death were unmistakable. When I proudly flaunted my knife to the girls, they showed no interest. Thinking, perhaps, Aunt Getel would appreciate my new possession, I tugged at her slip to rouse her, but she wouldn't budge. Finally, I screamed in her ear as loudly as I could, "Aunt Getel! Wake up! Look at what my mama stole for me!"

Dully opening her eyes half way, she slurred, "Wha' did she sshteal?"

At that precise moment, a shadow fell over me. As I glanced up, my mother slapped me across the face with such savagery that I went flying halfway across the kitchen floor. I lay there stunned, tears cascading down my cheeks. The entire right side of my face was burning, and blood was pouring out of my mouth. I felt around with my tongue, and found that my two front teeth were gone: another conspicuous difference that gave my classmates more ammunition with which to ridicule me.

There was nowhere to hide, so I crawled to my urine-stained pallet, covered myself with my scratchy, olive-drab colored wool blanket, and sobbed for a very long time. I had learned my lesson: You can steal, but you never squeal.

I never saw my Swiss Army knife again, and my mother never took me back to Woolworth's. And it was at least three months before I could hear again out of my right ear.

◄∿►

My Aunt Getel died about six months after she moved in with us. For the last three of those months, she was a living cadaver reeking of gangrenous flesh. Decades later, I realized, during a return visit to Cleveland, that the smell of her dying had burnt itself forever into my subconscious. Out of curiosity, I drove over to the East Side to see if our faded tenement was still standing. It was, and, as ugly and neglected as always, it was still teeming with life. I couldn't resist going inside and starting up the stairs, still dark and trash-strewn. When I reached the sixth-floor stairway, I swear, Getel's smell was still there. I turned and left.

◄∿►

Two weeks after the knife fiasco, just as I was getting settled in my desk, I wet my pants. I never even felt it coming out. It was suddenly just there, and just as suddenly, two or three times a week. Had it not been for the awful odor, I'm sure no one would have known of my secret torment. On occasion, the putrid stench of stale urine would be so insufferable in that poorly ventilated, third grade classroom that Miss Green, after shushing the "P.U.s" and "Phew, he stinks," would exile me to the coat closet or send me home with a note pinned to my shirt which, out of fear, I always crumpled up and threw away.

If I had any self-esteem at all at the time, it was soon gone. My sadistic and heartless classmates, one and all, because of my impudent bladder, shunned and ridiculed me. They were impressively skilled in the art of childhood cruelty. During recess and lunch, I, alone, would shuffle aimlessly around the grass fringes of the playground or perch on the monkey bars where, with head bowed and hands-in-pockets, I would sneak glances at all those cruel and inhuman children scattered everywhere, clowning around, skipping rope, flaunting their yo-yo virtuosity, or playing catch, hopscotch, marbles, tag, and jackstones. I was never asked to anyone's house after school to play, and I never got invited to sleepovers or birthday parties. And that year, I only received one Valentine, from Rosalyn Rabinowitz, who had had the misfortune to pick my name out of a hat.

Every day after the final, jarring bell reverberated through the labyrinthine hallways and silence, calm, and shadows swapped places with the glare and pandemonium of the school day, I would walk home—alone—sit on the curb and wait for the rabbi's assistant to drive up in his racketing junk heap of a "Woodie" and take me and a handful of other Orthodox Jewish boys from the neighborhood to the malodorous *heder*, where no one ever took notice of my stench.

To complicate matters, I would, on occasion, wet my bed as well. When my mother first discovered the soiled sheets, she said nothing. It apparently never entered her mind that, perhaps, I was physically ill. For some reason, when it came to her children, she seemed to have no parental sympathies.

After a few weeks, however, my mother decided she would personally cure me of my bed-wetting, and she did. It turned out to be a bittersweet cure in that I received a hell of a lot of attention, but at the expense of having to sit stark naked in a frigid tub of water.

I vividly remember her lifting me from my wet pallet in the middle of the night, removing my underwear, and practically tossing me into the tub of ice-cold water. As I sat there wide-eyed and terror-stricken, rocking to and fro with my hands desperately clasped to my bent knees, she would sit on the toilet seat watching and shrieking over and over, "How could a young boy be so lazy, not to pish in the toilet? Such a disgrace! What are you? A *shvartze*!"

Not even the staccato clacking of my teeth, nor the violent shivering of my body, nor the rivers of tears that flowed without pause down my deathly pale cheeks before dropping into the bath water softened her heart.

I have no idea where she came up with that treatment, but, thankfully, after six or seven of those insufferable baptisms, I was cured. It took years, however, before my classmates stopped calling me "Stinky." And it seemed like forever before Miss Green stopped asking me in front of everyone at least twice a day, "James, do you need to piddle?"

BEDLAM

I needed desperately to lie down.

The door of the shithouse led straight into a cramped dormitory of 30 or so graffitied bunk beds—some wood, some metal, all in disrepair, and all occupied except for one bottom bunk. The beds were arranged in haphazard rows with barely a foot or so of space between them.

I lay down with a sigh on the stained, lumpish mattress of the empty bunk. It sagged so much, I felt as if I were suspended in a hammock. There were no sheets or pillows, so I rolled a coarse, scratchy, army blanket I found under the bed into a cylinder to rest my head on.

As consumed as I was, I couldn't sleep. I have never been able to fall asleep in a lighted room, and lights were everywhere here. The dorm was separated from an adjoining rec room by a portable, accordion-like partition that missed the ceiling by a good four feet. As a result, the flickering lights of the rec room lit up half the dorm. There was also a lighted, overhead bulb in a metal cage, just above the partition nearest my bed that was never switched off, as were the yellowish lights that streamed through the door of the shithouse.

Outside, the Klieg light swept its intensely dazzling rays through the windows and across the dorm exactly every 60 seconds. It was so light, you could read fine print. In fact, I could clearly see on one of the bed slats above me the hand-carved sentiments, "FUCK THIS PLACE!"

The noise, too, kept me awake, alert, on edge. The reverberating, dissonant sounds of sleeping prisoners—groaning, moaning, wheezing, coughing, talking, snoring, farting—along with the continued all-night march to the shithouse became magnified, and, after awhile, maddening. Then there were the sounds of those still awake and active in the rec room that passed through and over the cheap, thin room divider—a turbulence of talk, laughter, and anger punctuated by an occasional poignant whimper and the fleeting clack of a billiard ball. And above all this was the constant ticking of the wall clocks and the throbbing and thumping of ancient, ailing, overworked heating units.

The light, the noise, and also the stench—the suffocating stench of putrid bodies, cigarette smoke, halitosis, and human gas that blended with the shithouse smells—kept me from what I needed most, the escape of sleep.

So I lay there with eyes wide open in a state of maniacal angst. After about 15 minutes, I got up and walked over to the other side of the partition. It was 5 a.m., yet the room was in full swing, swarming with sweating, animated, restless, prisoners; all without shirts, and some without pants due to the oppressive heat. There were boom boxes of every size everywhere—on the floor, on the chairs, on the tables, and on bare, black shoulders—blasting out simultaneously, hard rock, Afro-beat, funk and the crude, staccato lyrics of rap. This, along with a babble of talking, arguing, and TV noise, was altogether deafening.

In the middle of the room, which was about half the size of a high school gymnasium, four cocky, bantam-sized Puerto Rican caballeros with white handkerchiefs knotted around their foreheads and smoldering cheroots in the corners of their mouths were strutting around a broken down, slightly listing pool table. Every so often one would hawk out a mess of tobacco-stained saliva onto the cigarette butt-strewn floor.

Three wobbly card tables were occupied solely by blacks playing some sort of rummy game. The black contingent, which is to say the majority, also had exclusive rights to an old, black and white, Magnavox TV with a set of rabbit ears coupled to a coat hanger for better reception. The TV stood in one corner along with a dozen or so metal chairs, all occupied by blacks. In another corner of the room, a group of wiry blacks with well defined muscles was running through a succession of karate drills wearing nothing but filthy Jockey's and headbands.

None of the whites, of which there were only a few, were conversing or participating in "group" recreation. They were either standing watching TV behind the seated blacks, or sitting alone on the floor against the walls. From a distance they looked like broken men, lost boys, subdued captive animals, suddenly at the mercy of the bigger lions and the lion tamers. Maybe, like me, they had no choice but to leave whatever misguided arrogance they once had on the other side of the fence, along with their dreams and aspirations.

MANNA (FROM HEAVEN)

The day after Aunt Getel died, my mother asked Regina and me to remove the sheets and blanket from her deathbed. As we tremulously set about our macabre task, we noted a prominent lump at the foot of the mattress. It turned out to be an old leather purse which, when lifted up burst open, exposing thick bundles of cash held together by rubber bands, string, or ribbons. It was so heavy, it dropped on the floor, sending an avalanche of silver dollars and smaller coins rolling across the pitted linoleum. Hearing the clatter, my mother ran into the room, seemingly ready to scold us for something, but upon seeing the bonanza on the floor, she froze. After staring stupidly at it with her mouth open for a moment, she got on her hands and knees and in a frenzy scooped up the coins into her folded apron. When she had gathered them all, she just sat there and cried.

Not knowing what to do, I instinctively walked up to her and hesitantly laid a hand on her shoulder. She looked up, smiled, took my hand off her shoulder, closed her eyes, and pressed her warm lips against my palm. I will always cherish that one soft, tender moment. Deep in my heart, though, I know it came not out of love for me, but rather for her serendipitous fortune.

The unexpected windfall, which we spent most of the morning counting on the kitchen table, added up to nearly eight thousand dollars. We never really found out, for sure, how Aunt Getel acquired such a bulging purse. The most plausible explanation was that she came by it, either legally or illegally, working as a maid for my father's brother-in-law some years before. He was a prominent gangster with ties to the Mafia and a part owner of the Mounds Club, a gambling house just outside the city limits.

In any event, my mother used the money to purchase half of a duplex in Cleveland Heights, a blue-collar neighborhood just southeast of the greater city which, for some reason, had become home to many of the Jews who had had the good fortune to escape the urban ghettos and the African-Americans who had been steadily following them.

The particular street we moved to, however, Derbyshire Road, was devoid of Jews. We became the first. There were many children in the neighborhood, mostly Catholics, who would have nothing to do with the Scheiner kids—other than launch attacks with their fists, open fire with stones or snowballs, or besiege us with ethnic slurs and derogatory names. It was at those times, I would close my eyes and pray that we would all go back to the tenement to be among our own people.

My cousin Esther didn't come with us. That's all my parents needed—one more kid. I think they put her in an orphanage. We never heard from her again.

The other side of the duplex was purchased by my mother's older sister, Ruth, whose husband, Shlomo, although a tough-looking ox of a man, proved to be as much a milksop as my father. A corrupt, immoral simpleton in Poland, he had wandered like a gypsy among the various Jewish settlements hawking housewares out of a horse cart. In Cleveland, however, he somehow learned to drive and became an American huckster. He got hold of a banged-up Ford panel truck which he would load up with cheap rolls of linoleum and peddle them door-to-door to the trusting farmers in the Ohio and Pennsylvania countryside with the promise, of course, to return in a day or so to lay it on their floors. But once they paid him, he never showed up again.

His road trips usually lasted a few days, during which he slept in the truck. On occasion, however, usually following one of his frequent knock-down, drag-out squabbles with Ruth, he would disappear for months at a time. We suspected that he spent those prolonged absences either locked up in a slammer, somewhere out in the sticks, or with another woman.

They had one child, Rosalyn, a sloe-eyed moppet with curly, raven-black hair, a peaches-and-cream complexion, and a Roman profile, but possessed of a most repugnant personality. A selfish, spoiled, stuck-up brat, she was the very model of a Jewish-American Princess. To make matters worse, my mother, who never showed *us* love and tenderness, made no secret of her affection for this snooty cutie by adding a seemingly endless succession of gifts of clothes and jewelry to her burgeoning treasure trove, including a gold, Bulova watch on her tenth birthday.

Regina and I detested Rosalyn. We were as envious of her as is humanly possible. Rosalyn knew it, loved it, and threw it in our faces every chance she got. We did, however, manage to even the score, more or less.

During one of our childish, snooping expeditions around our new house, Regina and I discovered that one of the casement windows that opened into the basement on my aunt's side of the house remained unlocked. That window soon became a door to a series of unsanctioned, clandestine adventures. After making sure no one was home by ringing the front doorbell, we would squeeze through the casement window, drop to the concrete floor, and sneak up to Rosalyn's room, or as we called it, "the gold mine," where, while I appropriated bubblegum and stuffed my pockets with assorted candy bars from an unbelievably well-stocked cache hidden in the closet, Regina would snoop around the bureau drawers and closet, fondle cashmeres and dresses, and, on occasion, model them.

We could never understand nor could we ever swallow my mother's unyielding fondness and devotion to Rosalyn, who she nicknamed Honey. We spent hours deliberating this puzzle, always ending up with the unthinkable. Perhaps Rosalyn was not Shlomo's daughter at all, but, rather, the product of a depraved liaison between our father (whom she resembled) and Aunt Ruth. We also concluded that our mother knew of all this, but, not wanting to expose a humiliating scandal and chance losing her "wage slave" husband, chose to shrug it off.

I was ten when Regina's and my most fervent prayer was answered. After one particularly bitter quarrel with Ruth, Uncle Shlomo ran out the front door, jumped into his battered truck and disappeared for good. After six months, Aunt Ruth took a Greyhound to Miami where, for the next 35 years, she waitressed at Wolfie's, as did Rosalyn after graduating from high school. Before leaving, however, she sold her side of the duplex to a young couple with three children. They were the first "coloreds" in the neighborhood. The number of windows that were then broken in our duplex increased immeasurably as did the racial and ethnic expletives and epithets. Within a year, however, the two colored boys next door who had suddenly become tall, mean, and strong, put a quick end to the hostilities by breaking the jaw and arm of the little bigoted monster who had dared call their little sister a "jigaboo" and had thrown her school books to the ground.

My mother, however, never addressed the anti-Semitic harassment, but, rather, treated it with calm indifference as if it were either something to be expected or fearing, if she complained, it might provoke greater displays of torment.

Within a year of moving to the suburbs, Regina found out, having overheard a late-night discussion between my parents, that our mother was once again expecting. The fact of it became rather provocative since she was pregnant with twins and wanted to have an abortion which, apparently, was of no concern to our father. The discussion, at any rate, was pointless since it took place years before Roe v. Wade. She went on to give birth to my youngest siblings, Arthur and Barbara.

A DREAM GONE WRONG

Aunt Getel's posthumous largess made possible my mother's dream—a bakery. She set it up on one side of a small, newly built, nondescript building on Taylor Road and called it "Honey's." On the other side was Harry's Delicatessen, owned by the landlord, a bald butterball with a dill pickle for a face who, even in winter, was invariably wet with and smelled of stale sweat.

Located in the heart of a burgeoning Jewish community, success appeared inevitable for the two ventures; but although Harry's was a gold mine from the start, Honey's was a bomb. There was certainly nothing wrong with the breads and pastries; it was just that there were already two flourishing Jewish bakeries, each less than a mile away.

Whatever possessed my mother to risk her life's savings and Aunt Getel's posthumous largesse on a third bakery in that neighborhood was beyond reason. What did she think she could offer that they couldn't? Perhaps, like so many fools eager to fulfill the American dream of owning one's business, her judgment became blinded and irrational.

So Honey's Bakery became a constant source of *tsuris*. It survived, albeit barely, however, due to the large quantities of bread and rolls Harry needed, and because, unlike the "9-to-6" hours of the competition, Honey's stayed open 24 hours a day, closing only during the High Holy Days and Passover. It also survived because I was pressed into service by my mother to clean the place and assist with the baking.

Gratis, of course. To further save on labor costs, Regina worked along-side my mother as a salesgirl.

Bakers bake at night, which meant that Friday after *heder*, I would grab whatever I could find to eat, go up to my room, try to sleep until ten, get dressed, and walk the mile and a half to the bakery. There, I would put on an apron, stand on a box, and mold huge mounds of dough into bread, rolls, and bagels.

For a while, it was fun playing with all that dough. Perhaps it took the place of the toys I never had. But then, when summer came, the shop, with its sweltering brick oven, became an oppressive furnace. Stinking and sticky from the streams of sweat, I found it a grueling physical and psychological grind. Every weekend for six years, I toiled all night Friday and all night Saturday. The other nights my father toiled in solitude. On Sunday nights, I usually went to the movies, hunkered down alone with a large box of popcorn. During the summers, Easter, and Christmas holidays, however, I worked every night.

Frustrated and defeated at the failure of her dream and not having a moment to call her own, my mother soon became more out of control than ever. She was forever bickering and quarreling with my father, often in front of customers, blaming him, of course, for her failure. "Maybe," she would shriek, "if the dreck you made was any good, people would buy!" The one-sided spats always ended with her marching off mumbling something about what a mistake she had made marrying a *shiker behaime* (drunken fool).

Right under our eyes, she aged. Her face became drawn and outrageously wrinkled. Dark shadows appeared under her puffy, reddened eyes and her hair, which she no longer bothered with, thinned and turned a dingy steel-gray. The only time she smiled or spoke gently was when she was waiting on customers. When the store was deserted, which was most of the time, she sat in a corner on a stool with a cigarette and just stared, suspended in some sort of dream state.

My father handled the sweat, the long hours, the emptiness, and my mother with bottle after bottle of J.T.S. Brown and pack after pack of Lucky Strikes. As for me, the ever-obedient, Jewish eldest son, there was nothing I could do but accept my fate.

Despite my insecurities and interpersonal immaturity, when I was 13, I was deemed mature enough according to the Talmud to undergo the rite of passage—the Bar Mitzvah—that would make me a full member of Jewish society. By the mere fact of having attended Hebrew school since the age of four, it was taken for granted that I was enlightened regarding morality, decency, devotion, justice, and, of course, religion. Somehow or other, I had become a "righteous man," able to assume responsibility for my actions, to say nothing of my bigotry.

Most Jewish boys look forward to this ritual ceremony, not because of its implications, but rather because of the party and gifts that follow the privilege of reading from the Torah at the Saturday morning service. It has become a phenomenon where not only the rich but also the not-so-rich beg, borrow, steal, and mortgage in an effort to make the occasion a Jewish "happening"—a tasteless, embarrassing, public spectacle of wealth, self-adulation, and pretentiousness. Parents spend fortunes in their thirst to surpass the garish "productions" their friends orchestrated when their sons became "men."

My Bar Mitzvah was an ethnic joke. I was an imposter—light years away from anyone's definition of physical and emotional maturity. I went through the ceremony at the synagogue, but because of our circumstances, there was no "happening," and no gifts. It was just as well, for who could I have invited? I had no friends in school. It became just another weekend. Before the ceremony, I had stayed up all night baking. When it was over, I slept, and then baked some more.

PRE-MED: MANDATORY MACHIAVELLIANISM

During the course of a college career—should one be blessed—he or she will meet up with a true educator, one who is not only knowledgeable and capable of creative thought, but also sincere, concerned, supportive, and morally sound. Such a person was my advisor, Professor Charles Alan Welch, then chairman of the Department of Zoology, later Dean of the College of Arts and Sciences at the University of Cincinnati. He was an unassuming man with a rather small, roundish head barely covered with wispy, reddish hair; numerous freckles, and a warm, charismatic smile. He was the paradigm of a true college professor and had over the years advised scores of pre-med students, such as myself, many of whom had subsequently become members of the faculty of the medical school.

At our first meeting, he immediately put me at ease.

"I chose zoology for you as your major, Jim," he said extending his hand. "Dean Hutchinson, over at the med school, tells me he prefers his applicants to major in that or chemistry. I thought zoo might be a bit easier though and if you do well, and I'm sure you will, during this first year, we can see about getting you a scholarship. There are many available for pre-med students. By the way, could you use a part-time job?"

Replenishing supplies and solutions for the labs, and caring for a colony of 500 or so albino rats that were the subjects of experimentation and martyrdom by the faculty and postgraduate students proved to be rather prosaic but rewarding work. It took every bit of six hours each week to complete my tasks; and I was paid $150 a month, which was quite enough for tuition and living expenses. The best part of the job was that it came with a master key.

My office, which soon became my primary home, was a sizable stockroom equipped with a refrigerator where I kept a supply of rations and a two-burner gas stove which I used to heat up Campbell's soup and make untold gallons of Lipton tea. Not infrequently, I would sleep on the large work table where I studied and made up solutions for the various labs.

During my first weeks there, I noticed several of the professors going in and out of a room down the hall from me. Late one night, out of curiosity, I tried the lock on its door with my master key. It fit perfectly, and I soon found myself in a small windowless room that contained nothing but a mimeograph machine set on a table, reams of paper, and a large metal wastebasket.

I couldn't help but poke around in the wastebasket heaped with inked stencils and unusable, smudged copies of memoranda, notices, schedules, experiments, and—to my great surprise—exams. Obviously, I added exploring that particular wastebasket to my daily routine and, as luck would have it, was able to get my hands on either a copy of or the stencil for just about every zoology exam I ever had to take. This, of course, accounted for my straight-A average in zoology.

The mimeograph room, however, was of no help to me in my other courses. I got a D on the first chem exam and a C- on my first English exam. I felt, for sure, I would soon be on my way back to Cleveland, doomed to a stale existence as a lunch-bucket worker in a dough factory.

While brooding over that funereal prospect on my way to the zoo building, a sudden intense fear took hold of me. My entire body began to tremble and although it was chilly, I was flushed with heat and sweat. Feeling faint and having difficulty catching my breath, I sat down on the grass. My heart was beating like crazy. After a few minutes, though, the attack passed, but it left me feeling empty, nauseated, and depressed for the next two days. I probably would have had more such panic attacks had it not been for Winny.

⌒⌒

The rat colony with its small dissecting laboratory was on the top floor of the Zoology Building, a four-story, garden-variety pile of bricks and stone that was usually forsaken at night except for me and, on occasion, a diabolical sprite by the name of Albert Winston Hotchkiss. Winny, as he insisted he be called, was a professor emeritus of biochemistry who spent most evenings injecting chemicals into rats and later cutting them open. While at work, he wore a long lab coat over immaculate Brooks Brothers' suits and a black beret on his mane of silver hair.

Winny was at least 70 years old, yet his mental faculties were worlds above mine. His hands, however, on occasion, trembled mercilessly which was why he often asked me to help him dissect the rats in order to see what effect, if any, the chemicals he had injected had had on their internal organs.

We soon became relaxed with each other. After he was finished with his experiments, we would drink tea and he would ramble on about all the unanswered dunning letters he had written over the years to the U.S. Public Health Laboratory and the NIH "demanding" they investigate the more than 200 substances, such as nicotine, found in the general environment, he had found induced cancer in rats.

It was during one such interlude that, just for the sake of conversation I asked, "Winny, what do you do when you're not working on your rats?"

He smiled and answered simply, "Trip."

"Trip? Whaddaya mean?"

"Well, it's sort of a psychical experience brought on by taking hallucinogenic drugs."

The year was 1953, and although at the time those bohemian libertines, Jack Kerouac and Allen Ginsberg, were boldly hyping the Beat Generation with its accent on sex and drugs, it was unknown to me. I had to ask Winny what he meant.

"They're chemicals that affect one's mood and way of thinking," he explained patiently, "yet, at the same time, are able to preserve alertness and orientation. In essence, Jim, they alter your perception of the world. There's a lot of 'em. They come from plants—mushrooms, cactus; nutmeg which, I hear, is a particular favorite of convicts, and even morning glory seeds. I've tried a lot of 'em, but the one I'm really partial to is a synthetic one called LSD. That stands for lysergic acid diethylamide. It has a powerful, but, rather unpredictable, effect on the mind—"

"Like what?" I asked, fascinated.

"It acts differently in different people. When I take it I feel euphoric but, on occasion, fearful, and my senses, especially visual, become intensified. Colors seem brighter and sometimes I get these kaleidoscopic illusions of geometric designs or I see beautiful or monstrous faces; animals, especially snakes, and landscapes. While on it, or, as they say, 'tripping,' I feel depersonalized. I feel as if I'm either within or without my body, or sometimes both. When within, there are all sorts of openings leading into alleys which I explore and which take me back in time to my childhood or to the future, and where I find myself with an intensified ability to concentrate. I start mulling over such philosophical, religious, and cosmological questions as to who I am, and what is this existence I'm in. It's really hard to describe. But actually, I use it for its after effects. You see, it wears off in about ten or 12 hours and then for a day or so I have a sensation of well-being and serenity. My head is clear . . . refreshed. Life appears in a new light. Food tastes better and everything is brighter. That's why they call the drug California Sunshine. It's as if I'm . . . well . . . at home! It's truly a mystical experience. But don't you dare try it, son. Not now, anyhow, while you're in school."

"How'd you know about this stuff?" I asked him, shaking my head.

"Well, you see, for years I've suffered from depression. So bad at times I've even tried to commit suicide. Once, when I was in a private sanatorium near Los Angeles, my psychiatrist was experimenting with LSD in his patients with depression. Because of its euphoric potential, he was using it as a psychotherapeutic agent, just like Valium or Thorazine, but he also believed the drug had the ability to produce a state of mind that in and of itself resolved psychological problems. Frankly, it never really worked well for me, but I enjoyed it! I think, though, it's the cause of my hands shaking. Anyhow, you stay away from it!"

As it turned out, not too long after my panic attack, I did enter Winny's world. It was the night after that damned D in chemistry. I was feeding the colony, feeling like shit and so demoralized and upset, I couldn't get myself to study for a history exam in the morning. I was almost finished with my task when Winny shuffled in sparkling with serenity.

"What's wrong?" he rumbled when I despondently raised my hand in greeting, "You look like a basket case."

"Ech! I got a D on my chem exam. It's over, Winny! I can't do it. I'm gonna hafta go back to that fuckin' bakery!"

Suddenly morose, he studied me for a while, then snapped, "Wait here! Don't panic just yet! Jimmy, I have just the ticket for ya!"

After a half hour he returned, smiling complacently as he pressed a couple of small, heart-shaped, peach-colored pills in my hand and urged, "Here! Take one of these before you study."

"They're not that LSD, are they?"

"No. Don't be afraid. You can trust me, can't you?" he murmured softly noting my reluctance. "They're 'bennies.'"

"Bennies?"

"Yeah. Benzedrine. Speed. They'll make sure you do **OK**. Trust me. They expand the capabilities of your brain, kind o' bring out its potential."

I thanked him uncertainly and went down to the stockroom, brewed a flask of tea, and vacillated about taking the pill. *What*, I fretted, *if they are LSD?*, but then as I impulsively gulped one down I thought, *Oh, hell, what've I got to lose?*

Within minutes, an insidious, titillating impulse unfurled itself throughout my brain, forging an intoxicating blend of confidence, euphoria, and warmth. Suddenly, I became an energetic, eager, excited, and focused scholar. I felt, for the first time in my life, truly alive.

Winny was ecstatic over the quantum leap in my grades and, of course and rightly so, took full credit. Knowing I would need more— a lot more—of the wonder drug, he arranged with a "source," a pre-med student on a basketball scholarship, to attend to my needs.

At the end of my freshman year, Dr. Welch called me into his office to congratulate me on my 3.75 average. "Not bad for a guy who was admitted here on probation," he proclaimed. "I'm real proud of you, son."

CON JOB

Throughout the years, I have often been asked why I chose to become a doctor. It was not because of any of the traditional whys and wherefores. There weren't any firm, family traditions, well-meaning parents, or virtuous role models to coax or rouse an interest in medicine. Nor were there any decisive incidents that might have inspired such a vocation, like, perhaps, a life-threatening illness or some sort of crippling injury. I was never piqued by scientific matters. I knew nothing of such lofty philosophical abstractions as altruism, humanitarianism, or idealism.

As it turned out, it was my bitterly frustrated mother who was the *agent provocateur* of my choosing the field of medicine. In fact, I had no choice in the matter.

Intent and unshakable in her resolve to overcome her blighted hopes, my mother saw me as her savior and brainwashed me with such thoroughness over the years that I could never imagine being anything but a doctor. With remarkable cleverness, she made a compelling case—the *gelt*, the respect, the big house, the big car, the big this and the big that.

"You see, Yosele," she would say to me, "to be a doctor is golden. That's why I'm working so hard: for you. So you can go to college and be a doctor and have a big car, and a big house, and go places. You'll be so rich; you'll be able to take care of me when I'm too old to work anymore. You'll have such a big house, and there will be room for all of us."

Unfortunately, in a profession where emotional maturity is a prime educational objective, I never had the chance to purge myself of the outrageously immature and unsophisticated motives that had paved my way into it. During medical school, my personal maturity was retarded by my social isolation in the classroom and on the wards of the hospital: an isolation that was an epilogue to that of my childhood and adolescence. And throughout my residency it was retarded by the time and effort spent in my struggle to cultivate and adopt the physician's role and image. As a result, I had no time to establish a personal identity or to resolve my emotional problems, especially when confronted through it all by an abusiveness that echoed the atmosphere and circumstances of my childhood. Thus, hopelessly and irretrievably entangled in my subconscious, exalted image, I was determined to become an "M-Deity."

INQUISITION

For the first time in the history of the med school, the powers that be were interviewing all applicants considered especially promising before deciding on whether or not to admit them. Of the 40 or so pre-meds in my class, only 15 had received invitations for interviews. Of these, two or three were women. Six were Jews; I was one of them.

No one knew what to expect in the way of questions or what impact the "inquisition," as it was soon labeled and heralded by the Jewish crowd, would have on the overall selection process. My new friend, Malcolm, who worked at the dispensary, expressed one assumption: "The bastards just wanna see what color we are and what our noses look like. I heard they might even take a look at our *putzes*."

In truth, his bitter harangue wasn't too far-fetched, inasmuch as every college of medicine in America had an unwritten, unspoken, but very much implied "internal quota system." It was a cold, hard fact every Jew and every Negro and every woman aspiring to be a physician was well acquainted with. It wasn't that being a member of a minority group, "except, maybe," those in the white medical establishment claimed, "when it came to Negroes," made one unsuitable to practice medicine, but there were always those—from the dean on down—who were egregious racists, sexists, or anti-Semites, who took extraordinary pains to keep such "elements" to a minimum or, even better, out.

So to us Jews, the notion of a personal interview given by, as the whisper went, a clique of smug, sanctimonious, God-fearing, Christian snobs fired up nightmares of mental suffering regardless of how impressive one's educational achievements had been or how well connected one was. It stood to reason that many, perhaps most, of us therefore didn't stand much of a chance of being accepted. As Malcolm so aptly wailed one night when I went down to the dispensary to pick up a fresh supply of bennies, "It's just gonna be a fuckin' waste o' time. I heard from my dad—you know he's a surgeon in Toledo—that the dean and the rest of his *tuchis*-lickers were nothin' but a bunch o' fuckin' bigots!"

I, perhaps, was the most scared of all, inasmuch as my expository faculties, not to mention my social skills, were, to say the least, inept. Other than to Winny, I had rarely, if ever, expressed my sentiments or convictions, and having never done anything out of the ordinary, notwithstanding my unearned 3.75 GPA, I knew it was going to take nothing less than an Academy Award performance to get past this hurdle. But it was one I was able to psych myself up for, thanks to my invincible wonder-working friend Benzedrine who, I had no doubts, would see me through.

Every day until the morning of the interview, I rehearsed my script as if I were a matinee idol. Again and again, I recited my lines, hamming them up in the shower, at the table, or in front of the bathroom mirror.

At precisely 11:30 a.m. on a stormy, November morning—clean shaven, subtly scented with Old Spice, and decked out in a new, navy-blue, pinstripe suit and well polished Florsheim's—I gently tapped on the door of a small, muggy, windowless room in the basement of the med school. Beneath all my window dressing, however, was a frightened, quivering mass of goose bumps, butterflies, cold sweat, cold feet, and an awful lot of dyspepsia. *What if, by chance, I screwed up the interview, and didn't get accepted, what then? What the hell does one do with a major in 'zoo?' Teach? God, I couldn't stand that!*

After hearing a barely audible, "C'mon in," and while desperately trying to still my shaking hand, the quaking in my shoes, and the palpitations in my chest, I meekly opened the door. Cramped at a small table were two frosty, tweed-jacketed, bow-tied, professorial types.

Eschewing the usual civilities, one of the set looked up at me, squinted, and then, with a long, spidery finger, pointed to the lone chair across from him. I sat down, breathing hard with trepidation.

"Young man," he said testily, "what makes you think you belong here?"

Suddenly, for some reason, perhaps insecurity, I had an incredible urge to walk out. The thought of having to teach or having to go back to punching dough in the bakery, however, held me back. I smiled, looked him straight in the eye and told him exactly what he wanted to hear, calmly and with all the humility I could muster.

"Sir, I belong here because, to me, medicine is the most important, and far and away, the most exciting field of endeavor in our society, and I truly believe I possess the essential faculties, talents, and temperaments indispensable to becoming a competent, if not accomplished, physician."

"And what are *they*?"

"I am compulsive, persevering, exacting to the point of perfectionism, and highly inquisitive. I am also assertive, but not obtrusive, compassionate, and morally sound. I am also quite conscious of the fact that the making of a physician is a long, rigid, and intense undertaking. In fact, I read somewhere that it was an 'inflexible lifetime of commitment in a demanding and threatening environment,' but one, sir, I can emphatically, and with all confidence assure you, I have absolutely no qualms about entering. I feel confident that should my notion of becoming a physician become not a dream but a reality, I will be able to make a contribution to our society."

"Good answer, son," the cold fish effetely whispered with just a hint of a smile and a nod as his annoyingly mute sidekick kept on thumbing through my file. "All right then, tell me, since, according to your educational dossier, you haven't yet met with failure, how would such a dilemma affect you in your practice of medicine, assuming your dream does become a reality?"

It was a ticklish question, one that I had prepared for and rehearsed.

"Well sir, as you know, not only failure, but uncertainty, mistakes, and even death are unfortunately inherent in the field of medicine. Even with the current state of the art, there are still many unanswered questions and so much frustration, but thankfully less with each passing year. But, I'm sure, I don't have to tell you, there is still much to be done . . . much to learn . . . and, please, excuse the tired cliché . . . many mountains yet to climb. When one appreciates that there are, indeed, inherent limitations in the practice, or shall I say, the art of medicine, then one can prepare himself to deal with the frustrations, the risks, the gambles, the unpredictabilities, and the disappointments that are, thus, inescapable. Please, allow me to give you a personal example."

"As you wish."

With practiced gravity, I acquainted him with a conveniently fictionalized version of Aunt Getel.

"When I was . . . oh . . . six or seven, my aunt, a beautiful, innocent, terribly bright, young woman in her thirties came to live with us. Well . . . the truth of it was, she really came to die. You see, within a few months after her arrival to this country from Europe— Poland—and shortly after she had enrolled at Western Reserve to take up architecture, she had the devastating misfortune of developing cancer . . . breast. She was seen at the Crile Clinic in Cleveland where the doctors felt she needed a radical mastectomy. Within weeks following her surgery and a course of radiation, it was discovered that the cancer had spread to her liver and bones. There was now absolutely nothing anyone could do but pray."

Dripping with *schmaltz*, dewy-eyed, and mawkish as hell, I said I truly believed that my interest in medicine was kindled by that tragic affair.

Finally lightening up, the old professor broke into a smile, shook his head, and exclaimed, "You know, Mr. . . . . Scheiner, is it? As young as you are, you do seem to have a decent grasp and awareness of the profession. Very good. Yes, indeed! Now! Tell me, what have you been reading?"

"I just finished Morton Thompson's, *Not as a Stranger*, which I found . . ."

It was exactly 12 noon when I walked out of that little theater as confident about anything as I'd ever been in my life. I knew my performance had been a "solid sock" and a sensational testimony to the magical powers of Benzedrine.

MEDICAL SCHOOL: THE REALM
OF THE MARQUIS DE SADE

The most intimidating, demoralizing, and exhausting of all the required courses during the pre-clinical years is anatomy. There is a Herculean volume of material to commit to short-term memory, soon, if not immediately, to be forgotten.

The whole of the top floor of the medical school was taken up by the anatomy lab, and though girded on three sides by a procession of enormous, but small-paned windows, it remained dim, shadowy, and depressing. It was a vast chamber, yet contained nothing but a few scattered stools and 30, timeworn, dissecting tables in three, precise, parallel rows. Each table was like a coffin containing a gunny-shrouded corpse marinating in a pungent pool of formaldehyde.

Ordinarily, each cadaver was manned by four students, two to a side, but, since there were 97 students in the class, one of the cadavers had only three—Table 13. My table. The other members of my "coffin corps" were Jacob from Baltimore, the son of a Russian immigrant who sold men's suits during the day and large appliances at Montgomery Wards during the evenings to put his son through school; and Miriam, a mousey, disheveled, intellectual from Philadelphia who was bent on becoming the country's first female urologist. Malcolm was nowhere to be seen.

The three of us, thrown together by force of circumstance, somehow hit it off right from the start. Perhaps it was due to our collective Jewishness; but more than likely, it was simply that in order to get through this nightmare known as anatomy, we all knew there was no option but for us to work harmoniously as a team. So, the "Jewish Troika," as we called ourselves, became inseparable.

We studied day and night, lived in the library, snacked on vending-machine *schlock*, and whenever possible, crashed or bathed in our *pieds-a-terre*. Mine was a $10-a-week kennel in the attic of a seedy firetrap that probably should have been condemned during the First World War.

Being the good Jews that we were, we took a breather on Saturdays—well . . . Saturday nights, anyhow—down at Doctor Jekyll's, soaking up schooners of "fluids and electrolytes"—medical jargon for beer—with the rest of the class. We were there with only one thought in mind: to mellow out and forget, at least for a few hours, the hell we were going through. The next morning, however, when we awoke bleary-eyed, fuzzy-mouthed, and big headed, we remembered, with regret.

Neither Jacob nor I proved to be adept at dissecting our assigned cadaver, whom we nicknamed "the Marquis de Sade." Miriam, however, had incredibly talented hands. Whereas nearly everyone else hacked, slashed, chopped, or otherwise butchered their cadavers, her gentle, patient, meticulous dissections expedited by her long, delicate fingers were indistinguishable from those pictured in our anatomy text.

None of us will ever forget that first anatomy exam—the head and neck—probably the toughest regions of the body to grasp. God, we were scared! We stayed up all night sweating our brains with the Marquis, and, as luck would have it, we all passed.

Passing that first "sweat" disburdened us of an enormous psychological barrier. Now, we knew we could do "it," and we did. The troika, however, disbanded soon after the anatomy final. Jacob met a divorced nursing student over at Jekyll's and ended up living with her. Miriam and I, however, became each other's first lover and continued our liaison. Both of us, being superstitious, were fearful that if we parted company our grades would suffer; but more than that, we discovered that an occasional "flesh session" helped ease the angst of our lives.

During the first two years, a number of students either dropped out or flunked out—including one girl who found herself pregnant. None, however, of the 89 survivors remained unscathed. The thin got thinner; the overweight got underweight; the pale got paler; regular "monthlies" became irregular "monthlies"; those with glasses needed new glasses; those without got; and the once eager, sparkling eyes behind all those lenses gradually became dark and dulled; and no one finished with any fingernails to speak of.

Those having earned their freedom from the Stygian world of basic sciences were permitted to continue their martyrdom in the clinics, the wards, and in the emergency rooms of that wearied Grand Central Station known as Cincinnati General.

The transition from classroom to hospital was quite intimidating inasmuch as we, in our short, starched, white coats, suddenly became an intimate party to disease, suffering, and death. Even more traumatic, we became strikingly conspicuous. It was this high-profile visibility that placed us at a high risk for abuse.

During the clinical years, the class, by some mysterious means, was divided into teams of seven or eight students that rotated for three or four months at a time through the major medical specialties—surgery, medicine, pediatrics, ob/gyn, emergency medicine, and psychiatry. Time was also allocated for spending a few weeks in such specialized fields as orthopedics, urology, and ophthalmology. There was time, too, for a few electives, such as ENT which Miriam was keen on taking, if only to see if something could be done about her beaklike "schnozzola," as she called it.

"General" had become our classroom, and our teachers, the interns and residents. Under their tight-assed supervision we learned to examine, diagnose, and prescribe. But we paid for the privilege, not from our tuition, but through abuse of every conceivable kind—physical, verbal, sexual, ethnic, racial, and psychological. The idea was if you want to become a successful healer, you've got to learn to accept and tolerate the stress of hardship, adversity, and just plain, bad luck. Not only that, you must learn, during such trials, to mask your true feelings, and become a paradigm of grit and resolve.

Everyone, of course, knew of and anticipated this inescapable, denigrating rite of passage, knowing it to be, by design, fundamental to the cultivation of the macho identity physicians love to flaunt. What none of us knew, however, was that because of it, many of us would end up burnt out, physically or mentally ill, addicted, or dead, before even writing our first prescriptions. We would become martyrs to a training program flagrantly and inexcusably conducive to the creation of flawed physicians.

A MENACING VOICE

Finally accepting the delirium of my sleeplessness and the reality of this purgatory, I stepped forward to enter the room. Suddenly, over all the noise, someone shouted, "Welcome to Petersburg, Dr. Scheiner." Instantly, every head turned toward me, and every face glared at me, every boom box clicked off in sync. The contemptuousness of the voice was explicit. It came from a barefoot smart-ass-looking mulatto hunched over a cane wearing a grimy undershirt, shapeless pajama pants, and a Houston Astros baseball cap, ass-backward. He grinned at me, exposing a set of perfect, pure-white teeth; but his intense stare was charged with loathing.

When he saw me look at him, knowing I knew he was the source of this astonishing and improbable greeting, he raised his right hand above his head, and slowly clenched it into a defiant fist. Then he turned his back on me and with a conspicuous limp hobbled over to a small, black man, perhaps in his early thirties, who radiated danger.

I felt as if I had just been shot in the spine by a semiautomatic and had become paralyzed. I couldn't even blink my eyes or open my mouth or, for that matter, think, for as I stood there, trembling in that room's oppressive heat an overwhelming feeling of inescapable disaster overcame me. It was as if I was being swallowed by a black, turbulent sea of fear. *Who*, I tried to think, *was this tormentor who had just welcomed me to this place? How did he know who I was?* I knew I had seen his face before, but where?

I backed out of the room. I had nowhere to go but to the dorm and try, once again, to sleep. My bunk, however, had already been commandeered by another inmate, already asleep. There were no empty beds. In the corner by the windows I found a discarded blanket, filthy and practically in shreds, but I spread it on the floor and laid down on it. After staring out the windows at the falling snow, the distant stars and sliver of a moon, I closed my eyes and felt myself fall.

ANTOINE

In the summer of 1962 the barrios and slums of Houston were hot—not only from the heat of the sun, but also from the restlessness, discontent, and excitability of its inhabitants, many of whom carried guns, knives, and bastinados as if they were essential clothing accessories.

I'd begun my general surgical residency in July "26 on - 22 off" in the ER of the Jefferson Davis County Hospital, an ancient facility in which just about everything was either rundown, in disrepair, or discontinued. Although obsolete, it was probably the busiest hospital in Texas, which proved to be an intense training ground—grim, brutal, and exhausting. It was street theatre—a never-ending, chaotic, pulsating, head-splitting production with a varied cast of pathetic, disturbing, and, on occasion, poignant characters. Every hour of every day they walked in, limped in, wheeled in, or were carried in. Every age, every race, every color, and every religion in every manner of dress or undress imaginable surfaced at some time or other. And they waited and waited and waited: sitting, standing, sauntering, sleeping, or just staring. While waiting, a few died and a few were born on the beat-up, graffiti-scarred benches or in the toilets that stunk of sickness and death which no amount of disinfectant could ever wash away.

It was here that the casualties of the never-ending battles of urban warfare came, either to survive or to die. Their families, on the other hand, were being tested or undergoing treatment for the distinctive afflictions of their blighted lives: TB, syphilis, drug addiction, burns, rat bites, impetigo, and lead poisoning.

There was no let up: so many of them, so few of us. A leisurely lunch, a long coffee break, a finished cigarette, or a short nap were serious fantasies. There was no time to read, no time to question, and even less time to relax. And all that for a hundred bucks a week!

Every morning I had to shoulder my way through a crush of sick and injured people breathing down each other's necks within the small waiting room, and, after a lame nod to the decrepit pensioner guarding the jarring, mismatched double doors—which no one ever thought to repair or oil—enter the ER. There, I would be welcomed by a queue of gurneys holding those waiting to go to x-ray or journey up to the third floor to encounter the scalpels of impetuous neophyte surgeons who, in their quest for experience, would cut on anything or anyone, regardless.

Not surprisingly, I began to wake up annoyed, bitter, and resentful, and then, seeing what lay in store for me in that turbulent ER, I would sometimes explode. One such episode proved fateful.

I was a first-year resident rotating through the "bone service"—orthopedics. It was a Saturday morning and I was on rounds with the team. It had been an exceptionally busy night, with six admissions. One of the two "gun shots" that came in was Antoine Dubois, a defiant 16-year-old, who, while attempting to rob a liquor store had been shot with a .45 caliber, Colt semiautomatic by the owner, an army vet who had kept the "piece" as a Korean War souvenir. The bullet—a contraband, expanding dumdum—had entered the outer side of the kid's thigh just below the hip, where it made its distinctive, large, jagged, ugly entrance wound. It had then coursed through his thigh muscles, grinding them into hamburger, and then, still not finished with its havoc, shattered the shaft of his femur into a million pieces before finally coming to rest in his groin where it lay caressing the wildly beating, femoral artery.

It took most of the night to clean up Antoine's repugnant wound, and "hang" him up in traction in an effort to prevent his leg from shortening. At that time, the only treatment for his type of injury was months of traction, more months in a body cast, and then months of rehab. Continuous, intravenous antibiotics were also necessary to ward off infection—a catastrophic complication that, without their use, was almost inevitable in a wound contaminated by a dirty bullet and the dirty fragments of clothes it took with it during its vicious, supersonic trajectory. Amputation was certain should the bone itself become infected.

Since it was Saturday, everyone on the team except the guy on call wanted to get the hell out of there. So, after a cursory check of Antoine's massively, swollen thigh now encased in a second blood-soaked dressing, a perfunctory check of his traction, and a quick feel of his foot pulse, we moved on to the next victim of what we blithely called "the Houston chapter of the Friday Night Knife and Gun Club." As a nurse pulled the curtain to close off Antoine's cubicle from the 30 or so others in that crowded ward, without thinking, I blurted, "Just think, if it wasn't for the niggers and the spics, we wouldn't have anyone to practice on!" Antoine, I could see, had heard me; but, at the time, lying there like a prisoner in shackles, he was too indisposed to do anything about it.

CRAVINGS

An earsplitting whistle reverberated around the room setting nerves on edge. After a moment of relief it blew again, even louder, this time, joined by the dissonance of a hundred groaning, griping "cons" resenting this rude intrusion of their sleep, and two guards armed with clipboards and pens shouting orders. It could have been Auschwitz.

Glancing around, I spotted a caged clock on a wall. It was 4:30 a.m., and this sadistic ritual had to be the first body count of the day.

I had been only half asleep, suspended in that anxious twilight zone that knows no peace. I stood quickly, soon wide awake, not just from the glare or the noise, but from the fear of my cravings. Since the moment I had been cuffed and shackled, I had been on edge: dreading the inevitable, inescapable denouement of a decade of drugs.

Until now, there had always been another, getable dose of that "magical solution." There had always been something—a shot, a pill, a capsule, a suppository, a liquid—something! Something to chew, suck, lick, inject, or just shove up my ass—something, anything to thrust into my body to relieve the hunger and deter the unthinkable.

There *were* drugs here—all kinds, I could tell. The evidence was unmistakable. Those who had ravaged their bodies with stimulants shuffled around in a state of agitation and talkativeness. Others, in dreamlike states brought on by narcotics, revealed they were no longer here in this prison. They had been carried away to another place, a place I knew quite well. I considered asking around for a "hit" but was afraid of getting tainted drugs or toxic doses.

As I stood there in that prison dormitory, humiliated and frightened, waiting to be counted along with the other dregs of society, I realized I could not go lower. I was 45; my life was wasted; my physical body, violated and polluted; my mind, anguished and strung out; and my soul, almost in hell.

PRISCILLA

It was towards the end of September, and the smothering heat and sultriness of the Gulf Coast had at last departed. The leaves were starting to turn. My pride, or perhaps my arrogance, in having thus far survived my residency seemed to have re-energized my wasted body and spiritless mind. As a result, I was looking forward to my next rotation: a relatively benign tour in plastic surgery. But just before taking leave of my tour through purgatory, an undeniably portentous moment occurred that changed the rest of my life.

It was near midnight on a Friday evening and as usual the ER was packed and chaotic. Suddenly, a tiny Asian woman forced her way through the crowd, pushed aside the tough, heavy-set security guard stationed at the double doors and screamed into the treatment area, "My baby, she swallows Drano!" A limp three-year-old child was draped over her shoulder, motionless. Even from where I was standing—30 feet away—I could see that the child's mouth had been set on fire from the searing chemical. Her crimson-color lips were grotesquely swollen and blistered. Her huge black eyes were wide with terror. She was barely breathing; the swelling in her throat had all but closed off her airway. As I awkwardly leaned over the tiny bundle to perform an emergency "trach" in an effort to get some air into her lungs, a sudden lancinating pain flashed from the upper part of my back on the right side around to the front, and then into my groin. It lingered for a moment. Then it was gone.

My attempt to resuscitate the child proved futile. She died before I even made the incision. An autopsy revealed that the Drano had practically eaten away her esophagus and trachea and had oozed into her chest cavity, cauterizing her heart and lungs.

After closing the diaphanous lids over the toddler's unseeing eyes and covering her tiny, innocent face with the bed sheet, I glanced over at the mother standing with arms crossed at the foot of the gurney. She showed no visible signs of grief. She was just staring straight ahead, obviously in shock. I had her seen by the psychiatry resident who sensed she was considering taking her own life. He gave her a huge dose of Valium and then admitted her for observation, knowing full well that the worst for her was yet to come.

We had all faced such horrifying deaths before, but somehow this one was different. Everyone had been stunned into silence. The immunity to such tragedy that I had supposedly acquired had clearly abandoned me. Perhaps it had never been anything more than a façade, for when it was all over I went to the toilet, entered a stall, vomited, and then just stood there crying. God, I was sick. But there was no time for reflection or brooding. There were patients to see.

The adrenaline rush that such crises induce requires one to become so involved in the situation at hand that he or she is completely oblivious to everything else going on, including bodily functions. I gave no thought to the pain I'd experienced when bending over the child. Compared to the job at hand it hardly seemed important, and I had unconsciously dismissed it. It was not until several hours later, when I used the bathroom before leaving the ER, that I knew the pain was more than just a cramp: my urine was streaked with bright red blood. I shuddered with fear thinking, *Oh, God, I've got cancer.*

The colicky pain reappeared just as I opened the door to my room in the residents' quarters. It was excruciating and was accompanied by an urgent need to urinate. I knew then, that I had a kidney stone. I ran down to x-ray where one of the techs took a film of my abdomen. There was a stone wedged halfway down my right ureter.

My narcissism would not tolerate a show of personal weakness, so I was compelled to treat myself. I paged the nursing supervisor, an overweight woman named Priscilla, who seemed to be attracted to me. Within minutes of telling her of my dilemma she was at my door. When I let her in she gestured for me to lie down on the bed on my side. She then reached down into the pocket of her starched white uniform and removed a needle, a syringe, and an alcohol swab. Very proper and business-like, she lowered my pajama bottom, rubbed the top of my buttock with the alcohol swab, and proceeded to inject me with a slug of Demerol.

Within an instant my entire body became flushed with an exquisite, sensual feeling of warmth. As I closed my eyes to luxuriate in this new and extraordinary sensation, I experienced an astonishingly intense "rush"—an ecstatic, orgasmic intoxication that after a minute or so melted into a floating, dreamlike state of semi-consciousness. I didn't dare move for fear the calm and soothing would be no more. The anguishing scene with the Asian child melted away, forgotten. Reality and I had bid each other farewell.

Not only the pain, but all the anger, anxiety, fatigue, depression, and fear that had plagued me faded away. I rolled onto my back and opened my eyes. Priscilla was staring, amused by my metamorphosis. As I stared back at her I felt myself become sexually aroused. She walked over to the door and bolted it. Lifting her right leg onto a chair, she raised the skirt of her uniform, exposing a well-rounded thigh, and unhooked the snap of her garter belt. She then took the bottle of clear liquid from her pocket, pushed the same needle and syringe she had used on me through its rubber cap, withdrew several cc's of Demerol, and injected it into the front of her thigh. I heard her moan as she carefully removed all her clothing, folded it neatly on the chair, and slowly approached me.

COLD TURKEY

The count being right, we were given the green light to go for "groceries." Breakfast was served at 5 a.m. After lining up in something close to a single file, we were led out into the dark and bitter-cold prison quadrangle. As we trudged silently along the crisscrossed, graveled paths, snow crystals struck my face, melted, then ran like tears. Having no coat, I was shivering, my teeth chattering. My feet, in the thin, canvas slip-ons, quickly became water-soaked and numb.

After about ten minutes, we reached the huge, corrugated-metal Quonset that served as the main kitchen and mess room. It was warm inside, but the vast space—bright and sterile—was infused with the overpowering, stomach-turning odor of commercial disinfectant.

I loaded a time-worn, gray, plastic tray with what, at first glance, seemed to be a substantial breakfast good enough to eat, and sat down at an empty table. I stared at the steaming food for a few seconds, then cracked and peeled the shell from one of two hard-boiled eggs. The usually pearly-white white was scorched nut-brown over much of its ovoid surface. There was a burnt stellate-shaped cavity in its dried-out core. I left the other egg go to toy with a greasy slice of prison bacon (bologna) which I ultimately pushed aside. I finally made do with toast and a Styrofoam cup of vile-looking and even viler-tasting coffee.

We left the Quonset at exactly 5:30 a.m. By then the snow had stopped falling and the sun was just emerging over the horizon, its rays painting the retreating darkness with a kaleidoscopic blush of muted colors. Back at the dorm—exhausted, tired, and still hungry—I managed to find an abandoned, unmade, lower bunk. I sat down on it, removed my mud-soaked slip-ons and socks, and removed my shirt. I was hot, queasy, and achy. My nose was stopped up, my eyes watery, and my breathing suddenly short and painful. I wiped my eyes and forehead with the back of my hand which became sopping wet with tears and sweat, and lay down. As soon as my head touched the mattress, my mouth spontaneously gaped open, giving vent to long-drawn-out yawns, again and again for a long time.

Forgetting for a moment that I was an addict, I thought I was coming down with the flu as a result of tramping, virtually unclothed, in the frigid slush; but when I continued to yawn as if possessed, and when what, until then, had been a tolerable yearning suddenly became a rabid craving—so powerful and compelling that I would kill to feel normal again—I knew I was "coming down." The doors to that circus they call withdrawal had just opened up. I could only lay there in panic—tense, frightened, alone—for there was nothing I could do. I had to ride out this "twister" on my own—unaided, unattended. I tried desperately to sleep, hoping to let the horror run its course while I was insensible and far away, but it was not to be. I would have no calm or peace while the storm raged. I was falling from a tightrope, and there was no net beneath me.

Lunch and supper came and went. Weak and without appetite, except for a peculiar yearning for something sweet, I stayed either under or on top of the army blanket, depending on whether I was sweating or shivering. Even as the day passed into night, I couldn't sleep. Sometime, during the dead of night, when the gut-grinding craving had become more than I could bear, the cramps started. At first they were dull, gnawing waves, but soon they became white-capped breakers, and before the sun rose it was as if a great tsunami in all its fury was surging through my guts forcing out filth from both ends.

Wasted, I could hardly stand for the morning count. The "screw" taking the roll glanced curiously at me but said nothing. Why bother? Afterwards, I made my way to the bathroom, and after emptying my burning bladder, stood in front of the cracked mirror and stared. I had become a filthy, fetid damnation. My sunken eyes were bloodshot and their pupils were widely dilated like ship portholes. I could now see vividly what I had never seen before, nor wanted to see—a loser. Reflected in that fissured, marred glass was a miserable wretch without class or character: a liar, a thief, a coward, and a greasy junkie.

During the twilight of the second day of the "crash," I sensed someone close by. I opened my eyes to find Antoine Dubois standing at the foot of my bunk. "Well, look who's the patient now," he said, staring down at me. When our eyes met, he nodded, thrust out his lower lip, grinned, and burst out laughing. Then he limped away, the thump of his cane in sync with that of the throb behind my eyes.

After a few hours the cramps left my stomach only to find their way to the muscles of my lower back. That, the weakness, and the torment that entered my joints made it almost impossible to stand. Then my hands started trembling, and I could feel my heart race. The uncontrollable yawns became so powerful and drawn out, I thought my jaw would dislocate. But worst of all was the craving.

I was so restless and agitated I couldn't stay still in bed. When not tossing and turning in the small bunk, I would walk and walk; shuffling and dragging my heels, trying to exhaust myself into a sleep. Finally after two days of angst, dead on my feet, drained, yawning and craving, I sank into that now-gamy, filthy bed beneath that irritating, wool blanket and slept, but waking, again and again, sweating, shaking, and unhinged by vivid but unremembered nightmares. It was sleep terror without letup that only those who ever "used" know. Someone whacked the soles of my feet with the sharp edge of a plastic clipboard. "Get the fuck outta the sack, sleazebag!" It was 4:30 a.m., time for the first count.

Holding fast to the wooden post at the head of the bunk, I managed to swing my legs over the side and stand up. I had never felt so rotten—dizzy, feverish, agitated, trembling, twitching, shaking, shivering, shuddering, aching, grimacing, yawning, and craving—all at once. I was strung out, crazed, kinetic, and close to losing control. After the count, I roamed around like a rabid beast—half-animal, half-human—amongst the dregs and miscreants who had been up all night. Some were spellbound by Mickey Mouse on the TV; some had their heads buried, playing cards; some were busy discussing solutions for the problems of the world, while still others shot pool or stood alone, smoking and meditating. None, however, paid any attention to me. By this time, they all knew what I was going through, most, having at one time or another, condemned themselves to suffer the same torment and despair of withdrawal.

In the far corner of the holding room, sharing a joint with an unmistakable minion, was the man I had seen with Antoine on that first night. He looked at me and held up a finger beckoning me to wait. He handed the smoking stub of the joint to one of his "brothers," and walked over to where I was slumped against the wall.

"Got the sweats, huh? Looks like you could use a toke. Whatcha on?"

"Darvocet."

He shook his head. "Hmmmm. I can get some, but it would take a few days. You need something now."

"That's for sure."

"I got scag, blow, bennies. Angel dust?"

"What'll it cost? I have nothing, really."

He smiled. "Oh, we'll think of something."

I was about to come apart. I had to have something, anything, and was about to take him up on his proposal. But after a moment of soul-struggle, I looked my new-found patron square in the face, and said simply, "No thanks." He seemed strangely pleased by my rejection of his offer. He told me if I needed any help whatsoever to call on him. As he turned to leave, he said his name was Bobby. He said he already knew mine.

God, but I *did* need something. I was hurting bad, but I knew that only by crushing this evil, this depravity, this delinquency would I be able to salvage my life. This time—my last chance—I would not stumble. I would not be defeated. I would not disappoint.

HANNAH

In the 1960's the field of orthopedic surgery was still rather primitive, and of no real concern to those charged with putting together the medical school curriculum. In fact, during the entire four years of medical school only a few days were allotted to its study. Other than learning that orthopods, as they are known, took care of fractures and dislocations, and loved to play with plaster-of-Paris, the field remained a mystery to most students, and, as a result, never attracted many followers.

In view of the imperfect tools, implants, and techniques used in repairing bones and joints when I was a resident, technical errors and complications were extremely common. They were expected—and therefore accepted—not only among the residents, but the staff as well. We were all in this together. There was no cutthroat rivalry, and no one was getting fired or abused. For the first time since the start of my medical education, I found myself relaxed and unthreatened. I was actually enjoying myself. Not wanting this pleasant state of affairs to end or perhaps because, subconsciously, the tools and gadgetry of the trade took the place of the toys I never had as a kid, I switched to ortho.

General surgery residents at County were on the go day and night, 24/7, for there was no end to the emergencies and complications inherent in their line of work. The orthopedic service, in contrast, had nowhere near that kind of volume, and since most of the cases that required surgery could be scheduled at one's leisure, it left plenty of time for a life: that is, if you were married, which most of the residents were, or blessed with a relatively normal psyche. Unfortunately, I was neither. I was a non-entity when it came to men, and, even more so, with women. Without a life, I merely existed: dinners—alone; movies—alone; drinking—alone; TV—alone; and brooding—alone. Finally, able to afford what passed for a car, I occasionally drove over to one of those grungy, smelly, Galveston beaches, and got a little sun—alone.

I was lonely as hell and randy as hell. Of course, I shouldn't have been. The hospital was swarming with single women dying to hook up with a doctor, even a timid, 26-year-old resident like myself. I guess I didn't have the guts or confidence, or whatever it was I needed to ask any of them out.

During my plastic surgery rotation, however, after daydreaming, *ad nauseum*, about that salacious, opiate charade with Priscilla, I paged her, only to learn she'd been forced to resign after she was caught stealing narcotics.

With Miriam gone—she'd transferred to another med school in Philadelphia—and Priscilla now totally out of the picture, my loneliness and frustration increased. I needed a woman. Desperately. A woman to talk to. A woman to have sex with. I was willing to do anything for one, even, I pondered, get married. The word "love" never once came to mind. What did was Vietnam. I wanted no part of it.

That being the case, my urgency for a wife and even children was perhaps nothing more than a Machiavellian delusion to lessen my chances of being dispatched to that Southeast Asian quagmire.

So, I called Hannah, a nice Jewish girl I had dated briefly in med school. After all, I rationalized, she was an attractive, decent woman, who would surely make an exceptional wife and mother.

The moment she answered the phone, she took my breath away. Her voice and words seemed surreal for, inexplicably, she seemed delighted to hear from me.

"You sound great! How've you been and where are you and what are you doing and . . . why the all-of-a-sudden call?"

After telling her what was going on in my life, I sputtered, "Hannah, I miss you. Really . . . for a long time, and," I lied, "I do love you . . . very much. I do know that now. I think we should get married. That is, of course, if you do have some feelings for me. I promise I'll make you happy."

She agreed, without hesitation, as I'd suspected, to my impetuous proposal. I knew she'd always dreamed of being married to a doctor and had always longed to be able at last, to "keep up with the Joneses."

One month later, May 2, 1964, I stomped on a wine glass under the *chuppah* of the Isaac M. Wise Temple in Cincinnati. The following year, on March 20, 1965, our first son Erich was born. I never had to serve in Vietnam.

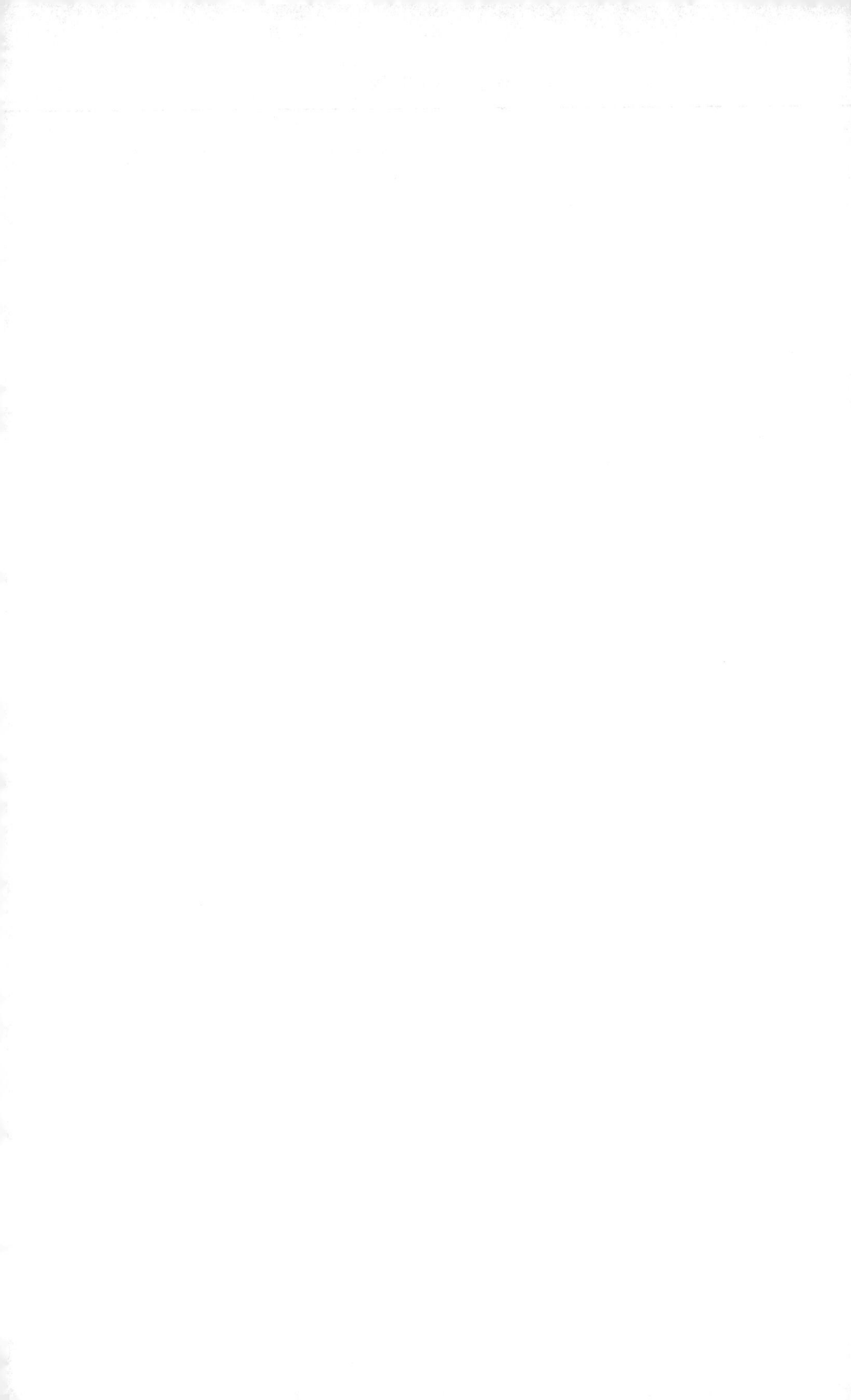

HANGING TOUGH

forced myself to march to the military-style Quonset hut for lunch—
two slices of margarined Wonder Bread and a container of milk, all
of which I vomited on the dirty, wet slush on the way back. In the
dormitory, on edge, tense, and strained, I still couldn't sit still. I had
to keep moving and wandered around. As the sun started to set I lay
down, closed my eyes, and had almost dozed off when suddenly my
right arm shot out like an errant missile, and then just as suddenly
snapped back, relaxed, and dropped on the bed. A few minutes later
it happened again, and then again and again; every time I closed my
eyes.

Towards morning, when my shoulder felt as if it had been
wrenched out of place, a similar boomeranging of both legs began
to occur along with a strange sensation. My legs felt as if an army
of small insects was eating away at them: tiny jaws pinching, pricking, piercing, gnawing, and crunching away under the skin and deep
within the muscles and bones. And then, my head began to jerk—
sideways. But despite my terror, realized I was actually "kicking the
habit."

Over the years, because of Hannah and the children, I'd tried on
several occasions to kick the habit cold turkey. But I never managed
to quite bring it off. The longest I lasted was barely two days. The
main obstacle for me was the unendurable hell of withdrawal. Now, I
knew, I had no choice but to go through it.

Somehow I made it through that third day, and I even slept—until jarred awake by the piercing screeching of a whistle, as usual, right in my ear. The count had begun.

"Everyone up! The warden's comin' thru."

When the warden stopped by my bed, he was apparently disturbed at what he saw. With a quizzical look, he studied me, then asked me if I was OK. "Sure," I said, "just hadn't slept in a few days. You know: strange bed, strange bedfellows."

"How long have you been here?"

"Four days, maybe."

"Do you need anything?"

I looked down. "Shoes." He glanced at my feet with their filthy, disintegrating slip-ons, shook his head, murmured something to the two guards who accompanied him, and walked on.

After we were "cut loose" by the guard with the whistle, I went to the bathroom. I looked at myself again in the mirror. Where once was a body, was an emaciated, sinister framework of bones. And where once was a head was a bearded skull with blackened bloodshot craters for eyes. My skin had turned a sickly ashen color, and my hair was graying. I had become the Marquis de Sade.

ANTI-SEMITISM

On June 30, 1968, my medical education was over. Thirteen years of consuming study, 4,749 sleepless or disturbed nights—over. Yet on that day, for me, there was no celebration, for there was no excitement. That delirious rush of mental intoxication at having surmounted a formidable obstacle was not there. In its stead was an oppressive awareness of desperation that would soon be followed, ironically, by 13 more years of anguish before coming to an end in, of all places, a federal penitentiary.

During the first three months of the last year of my residency, I and a junior resident had been given the honor of becoming personal scut-monkeys for the attending orthopedic staff at the Methodist Hospital who were, for the most part, a close-knit clique of self-worshipping, supercilious anti-Semites.

Almost immediately upon setting foot in that auspicious hospital, I sensed, hovering among the other diseases, anti-Semitism. For me, alone, there was no briefing and no introductions. I had to seek out the attendings to make myself known, and when I found them there was no firm handshake or a "welcome aboard." All I got after holding out my hand was a limp, finger-tip handshake, and, on occasion, out of the corner of a mouth a perfunctory quiver.

For three months, I examined and prepared their patients for surgery; stood, for hours on end, holding open surgical incisions with hoe-shaped instruments contemptuously known as idiot sticks until my fingers became rigid with pain, took care of the post-op necessities, did the paperwork; and, of course, massaged— non-stop—their egos, yet no one ever took the time to discuss his patients with me nor invite me for a cup of coffee. Although it is customary for the residents on a private rotation—as a gesture of thanks, for making the attendings lives much easier—to do at least their minor surgical cases, I alone, never once, had a scalpel put in my hands. I don't even recall ever being thanked. But I still gave it my best, even though my earnest efforts in caring for the patients of these members of the "old-boy network" of Texas medicine were neither acknowledged nor appreciated. These provincial Christians were not about to praise the efforts of an outsider, a "Jew-boy," let alone show any genuine consideration or courtesy.

Perhaps no one would have known I was Jewish, and the climate at Methodist would not have been so abusive had I not befriended Houston's busiest orthopedic surgeon, Dr. Bernard Bressler. When I first met him during a Yom Kippur service, a year or so before I came to Methodist, I had no idea who or what he was, but I was thrilled and honored when he later asked me to work for him. Hannah and I were newly married, and the $400 he paid me each month, for a few hours of work on weekends, was a real gift.

Originally from Brooklyn, Dr. Bressler had been in Houston for at least 20 years. He came to Houston because there was a large Jewish community there with lots of money, but without a Jewish orthopod. It was a golden opportunity since Jews prefer to be treated by their own. And he made the best of it. When I got there, he was still the only Jewish orthopod, but a lot richer. His money came primarily from the workmen's comp and personal injury cases referred to him by a host of greedy lawyers who specialized in such deceitfulness. These whiplash mavens and ambulance chasers loved him. And why not? He got their clients huge settlements by padding their medical bills with expensive, often-capricious lab tests, therapy, and surgery. He had learned early on how to make a fast buck by playing the litigation game—the higher the medicals, the higher the settlement.

Bressler had operated on thousands of spines. He cut open more backs in one year than most honest surgeons do in a decade. It was astounding how many people with bogus back pain would lie down on an operating table and go under his knife. They would submit to this surgery knowing full well they might wake up with *real* back pain or even paralysis, which some did. What mattered most to them was ripping off the insurance companies and being able to spend the rest of their lives as couch potatoes with fattened bank accounts.

Bressler was active on the staff of six hospitals, including Methodist, but hated going there because most of their orthopedists were (he didn't have to tell me) "jealous Jew-haters." With me working for him, he wouldn't have to go there—at least not on weekends. I would do his rounds on those days.

ELDORADO

Around the corner from the nurses' station in the orthopedic wing on the third floor at Methodist was a small, narrow kitchen which served as a stand-up coffee lounge for the staff. It also became the supply base for my drugs.

I had surreptitiously discovered this bountiful depository of drugs one night while on call. It was about 6:30 a.m. and I had just finished catheterizing a 92-year-old guy who had had his hip pinned the day before. By then, it was too late to go back to bed since I was due to scrub in the OR in a half hour. Needing a coffee, I went to the kitchen and poured myself a cup.

While standing there drinking and feeling, as usual, miserable, one of the nurse's aides came in holding a half-empty bottle of pills. She smiled, walked to the back of the kitchen, opened a drawer beneath the counter, and put them in. After she left, when I opened the drawer, I could hardly believe my eyes. There must have been 30 or 40 labeled bottles partially filled with a variety of narcotics that included Codeine, Demerol, Percodan, and Dilaudid. These were leftover meds that had been ordered but had not been entirely used by the patients during their hospital stay.

For the duration of my time at Methodist, this "coffee lounge" became my refuge; this stash, my "dirty little secret." These drugs helped me cope.

CHRISTMAS

After the warden's visit, I managed to slosh through the still-falling snow to the Quonset where I was able to wash down—and keep down—two, scorched, imploded eggs; toast, and a bowl of thick, tacky gruel, that may have been farina, with two cups of heavily sugared coffee. Afterwards I tried to sleep, but the jerking—although coming about less often and less intense—prevented me from doing so.

Later in the afternoon, as I laid there jerking, Bobby stopped by. He had apparently seen me eating well at breakfast and told me he was pleased that I was "making it." He suggested that I go down for Christmas supper, "best meal of the year." I was glad I did, because the turkey and trimmings were, in fact, good.

Afterward, before returning to the holding area, we were marched down to the dwarf's lair, where we received our Christmas presents: a change of underwear and socks, toothpaste, toothbrush, a box of Top's tobacco, and a small, thin envelope of cigarette paper. I asked about shoes but received no reply.

I was feeling better, but I smelled awful. I needed a shower, badly. The "shithouse" was empty except for someone standing in the shower with his prominent butt facing me. He was masturbating. I waited for him to finish and leave. I then stepped into the moldy, concrete stall. As I slowly showered with the barely trickling, lukewarm, rust-colored water, I watched the primeval cockroaches, silver fish, and an occasional centipede scurry about, pausing now and then to stare at me.

After drying and dressing, being careful where I stepped, I went to the TV. It had been commandeered by a wiry, gangling, sky-high black guy in his early twenties, who was either on speed, psychotic, had hyperthyroidism, some sort of attention deficit disorder, or all of the above. He was in a constant state of agitation. Over and over he jumped out of his chair to switch channels. With each show, he would rant, with a continuum of commentary, opinions, and criticisms. It made no difference what was on, he always had something scorching to say. I left the room and wandered aimlessly.

As I meandered, I saw nothing that even hinted of Christmas. The unwavering, dissonant scene continued to ebb and flow; its syncopated rhythm punctuated by frequent roulades of "motha-fuckas." No one but I seemed the least disheartened at being under lock and key for Christmas. For them, it was just another day. They seemed to be happy here—laughing, joking, chatting—presumably because whatever they had to face here was better than what they had to face on the outside.

Although Jewish, once Hannah and I had children, the essence of Christmas became an indispensable fact in our lives. The peace, the love, and the festivities of the state of mind that is Christmas, we found to be—as a family—extraordinarily contagious. Now, locked up, distant and apart, the joyousness had been replaced with melancholy. I needed to call home.

An unusually long column of touchy, impatient prisoners was waiting to use what was still left of the one, working telephone. A sign stenciled on the graffitied booth stated that all calls were subject to monitoring and were limited to ten minutes. No one paid any attention to this time limit. Consequently, the highly volatile queue became the scene of verbal and physical clashes. After standing in line for over two hours, I entered the booth. Although it was essentially unenclosed, it still reeked of human odors, cigarettes and marijuana.

The floor was covered with a generous heap of compacted trash and cigarette butts.

Hannah answered the phone. She had been crying. During the previous night as the boys slept, no doubt dreaming of presents and amusements, she had had a miscarriage. Just before dawn, she told me she flushed a perfectly formed, tiny body down the toilet. It was a three-month fetus—a girl. I hadn't even known Hannah was pregnant. In her anger, grief, and pain, she blamed me for this too. I was now, in addition to everything else, a murderer. Our conversation ended in less than five minutes.

I shook my head, went back to the dorm, sat down on an empty bunk, and clumsily rolled a cigarette from the "makings" I had received from the dwarf. I lit the crude, wrinkled cone, and deeply inhaled clouds of caustic smoke spiked with flecks of tobacco and paper that soon left my throat raw. After finishing my smoke, like everyone else, I carelessly flipped the lighted butt on the floor, knowing it could easily cause a fire. Then I stretched out on the bunk and fell instantly into a deep sleep.

HANNAH

My affiliation with Dr. Bressler came to an abrupt end when he learned negative rumors about me stemming from a run-in I'd had with a leading member of Houston's "medical brotherhood." Bressler said he was sorry, he wished me and "Hanela" well, but he couldn't take a chance on me. He advised me to "go as far away as possible" from Houston. I'd been blacklisted.

How could I tell Hannah? Her second pregnancy was turning out to be difficult, due to what Dr. Goldfarb, her ob/gyn, called "an incompetent cervix."

She had gone right to bed as the doctor had ordered and had stayed there except to go to the bathroom. But even so, the bleeding worsened. She was terrified. I called the junior resident to tell him what was going on and asked him to cover for me, and I drove Hannah, with my arm around her, to Dr. Goldfarb's.

On the way, I almost lost control of the Chieftain when she told me she was carrying twins! At first, we started to cry; but at a red light, when we had a chance to really look at each other, our tears suddenly changed to silly smiles. By the time we heard the jarring, blasting horns of the cars behind informing us that the light had changed, we were laughing jubilantly and somewhat out of control.

Dr. Goldfarb came right to the point, "I'm sorry," he sighed, "but the chance of a miscarriage is terribly real, here. We need to get you to the hospital ASAP."

As I frantically paced the waiting room, everything but Hannah and the twin fetuses within her womb now seemed inconsequential.

Realizing I was responsible for their well-being was especially fright-ening, given the reality of the situation which was: my residency was due to end in three weeks, I had nothing to look forward to, and I still hadn't had the nerve to tell Hannah about Bressler.

I drove home, popped three "percs," snorted "two-fingers" of Old Crow, set the alarm for 4:30, and called it a day.

When I awoke, I had a smoldering crater in my stomach and a magnificent migraine. I took another couple of percs with a glass of milk, and got ready for work. I had to make rounds. It was club-foot clinic day.

That clinic negated any relief the percs had afforded my headache, so before going up to the library to search the want ads listed in the back pages of the Journal of the American Medical Association, I took a couple more. There was only a single ad for an orthopedic surgeon. Some guy with an Italian sounding name in Arlington, Virginia, was looking for an associate. I phoned him. He was quite amiable, and once his questions regarding my educational background were out of the way, he asked, "So when can you come up for an interview? I'll be glad to pay the air fare."

"Next weekend, but only for one day since my wife is in the hos-pital. We're expecting twins!"

After hanging up I started to breathe a lot easier. I was sure he would take me on.

TRIUMPH

This time the sadistic whistle—despite its shrill, screeching turmoil rudely deployed at the very edge of my ear—was unable to wake me. I was too sick. It took the guard a few minutes to realize the fact, but eventually he silenced his whistle and sent for a doctor.

Three hours later, a sweating, bloated, old prison doctor nervously placed a frosted stethoscope on my chest and ordered me to breath with my mouth open: deeply. After listening, with his eyes squeezed shut, to a few breaths, he pulled out a huge, gold pocket watch, cupped it in his puffy hand, counted my pulse, and left without a word.

An hour later he returned with a gigantic, antiquated, hypodermic syringe equipped with an equally gigantic needle and filled with a huge dose of penicillin. He motioned to the guard to turn me over and lower my shorts, and then, without bothering to swab my skin with alcohol, plunged the needle deep into the muscle of my buttock. As he worked, I could hear his croaking breathing, and although he was behind me, I smelt his sour breath. His job completed, he instructed the guard to "throw" me in a cell, and left without a word. The guard then functioned as a clumsy crutch as I stumbled over to one of the cells just outside the holding area.

For the next two days, I lay under four coarse, woolen blankets curled up like a fetus on a filthy, thin, sheetless mattress on a narrow metal shelf hinged to the wall. When not spaced out and oblivious, I coughed bloodied pus with bits of gangrenous tissue out of my lungs into a succession of Styrofoam cups that came with the meal trays I barely acknowledged. Then the fever broke. The all-consuming, tormenting craving had at last come to an end. The "circus" was over.

DR. IANERELLA

Surviving on Big Macs, fries, and a tankerload of coffee, I drove non-stop except for an occasional snooze at rest stops, to Arlington, Virginia. With the last of our money, we rented a cheap, badly furnished, first-floor studio just off Glebe Road within view of the Pentagon.

The morning of my first day, I drove to the office, one of the modules in a small, stale, strip mall, excited, enthusiastic, and full of eagerness about the new job. I opened the glass door stenciled in boldface-black with the name—Salvatore P. Ianerella, M.D. A clanking bell secured to the top edge of the door announced my arrival. I closed the door as softly as I could. The cracked, stained walls of the waiting room were bare except for a small, handwritten sign next to the receptionist's window urging patients to check in with her first.

I went up to the sliding-glass window set in the far wall and watched for a while until the hatchet-faced receptionist finally twanged, "Yheas-s-s?"

When I told her who I was, she grudgingly managed to put down her book, stand up, point to a closed door on the right side of a narrow, short hallway, and tell me, "You can wait in there."

As she turned to return to her book, I asked her when the doctor would be in. She merely shrugged and said, "Who knows?"

I opened the door of the designated room, Ianerella's opulent office, and timidly sat down on one of the doctor's graceful chairs. Suddenly, feeling the need for something to alleviate my anxiety, I stood up and began to pace. Perhaps, I thought, letting my imagination run wild, a cup of coffee would help. I walked back out into the hall in search of a pot.

Besides the doctor's office and a vest-pocket toilet, there were three other rooms. The largest contained an old Picker x-ray machine—strictly no-tech. The other two were examining rooms—unadorned and austere.

There was no coffee to be found. Perhaps the receptionist could help, but I didn't have the stomach to ask her. Bored, I wandered into one of the exam rooms, and for a while stood over the medicine cabinet surveying the various instruments and supplies casually arranged on it. Aside from a reflex hammer, goniometer, and a prescription pad, there was a stainless-steel pan containing alcohol pledgets, assorted, disposable syringes and needles, and several bottles of injectables. One of them was all too familiar.

I picked it out of the pan with trembling fingers. It was a 30 cc, rubber-capped vial of Winthrop Laboratories' brand of meperidine hydrochloride—Demerol. Hearing voices and a door opening, I hurriedly replaced it in the pan and ran back out into the hall.

THE MANSION

"Get your things, Doc. They found a new home for you." It was the ferret.

I turned and noticed for the first time that the ferret had a name tag over his shirt pocket that read "Orville Taggert." He led me through a side door, out across the quadrangle, and through a heavily armed, barred gate onto a short path that led directly to what appeared to be a mirage.

Practically hidden between the razor-wired, garrisoned, south wall of the penitentiary and a forested tributary of the James River was a Federal Prison Camp. It didn't seem at all what one would expect of a prison: it was a two-storied, stuccoed, colonnaded building that may have been an ante-bellum, southern colonial.

The snow had melted, and I could see on either side of the once stately mansion expanses of grass crisscrossed by pebbled footpaths and framed by neatly trimmed boxwood. Behind the camp, leading down to the waterside was dense woodland. On the left, a gazebo lay rotting in the center of a well-worn running track, and on the right was a large, open shed overflowing with rusting iron plates, dumbbells, barbells, and weight-lifting benches.

The camp provided food, shelter, and a few amenities, along with a modicum of laxity and freedom, for prisoners either serving a short sentence for white-collar or execu-crime, of whom there were only a handful, or who, having behaved themselves while doing a prolonged stretch of hard time in more austere and punitive facilities were being rewarded by spending their last few months in the relative luxury of a FPC before returning to society.

As Orville Taggart and I walked down the path, I could see a small, tightly knit cluster of watch-capped men, with heads bowed from the wind, slowly jogging around the track. In the weight-shed, however, there were three or four shirtless, fanatical power lifters pumping iron.

The front door of the "mansion" opened into a small antechamber at the end of which a magnificently carved balustrade embraced a curved, oaken staircase. To the right of the staircase, the original partitioning, as well as the entire, outer wall where the new wing had been joined had been removed, making one spacious dormitory lined with neatly spaced, double-bunk beds. At the foot of each bed were two gray, metal, industrial lockers, some, with locks attached. To the left and behind the staircase was a doorless bathroom. It was spotless. The doorless rec room just to the left of the antechamber contained a TV, a couple of card tables, a dozen or so folding chairs, a Coke machine, and two intact, but graffitied telephone booths. The mansion appeared to be the antithesis of the holding area where I'd been up 'til then.

Taggert led the way to the second floor where the administrative and guards' offices were located. When he knocked on the door marked "FPC Administrator, Calvin Cavendish", there was no response. After waiting a moment, he gently cracked open the door and peered in. The administrator smiled and waved us in from his desk, behind which hung a large framed photo of President Jimmy Carter. Taggart placed my file on the desk and left the room.

The administrator was on the phone hard at work writing down a long list of groceries he was to buy on his way home. After a minute or two, he looked up at the ceiling, rolled his eyes, shook his head, put his hand over the receiver, and told me to sit down on one of the two, brown, folding metal chairs in front of his desk. I listened as he continued to chat about that evening's low-caloric, low-cholesterol, dinner menu. Finally, he said "good-bye, sweetie" and apologized for making me wait. He then stood up and came from behind his desk to shake my hand.

After the standard admonishments—no drugs . . . no weapons . . . strict silence during counts . . . no more than ten dollars and only in quarters in your pockets at any one time—he handed me a copy of the <u>FBP Rules for Inmates</u>, and advised me to "memorize it!" He then asked me if I liked to fish. Somewhat taken aback, I replied, "Not really."

"That's too bad. There's a river down the way loaded with carp—fun to catch, but you have to throw 'em back. Anyhow, if you decide to, we have some poles here you can use. 'Course, you'll have to dig up your own worms."

"Thanks. Maybe I'll try when it gets warm."

"Suit yourself. Let's go downstairs."

He assigned me an upper bunk at the far end of the dorm. "The black boys call this area Peckerwood Park," he whispered, "'cause only the white boys sleep in this section." He told me I had to have a job and hired me at 16¢ an hour to clean the bathroom. Before leaving, he ran his eyes over me and counseled, "Make up your bed neatly before seven, keep your person clean, your clothing tidy and in good order, and, remember, no one promised you a rose garden." He shook my hand, smiled and said, "I'm really sorry you're here, doctor."

DR. IANERELLA

Only three weeks after I started working in Sal Ianerella's office, he called me at home on a Sunday afternoon to let me know he was leaving that evening to attend the annual convention of the American Academy of Orthopaedic Surgeons in New Orleans. He said he would be gone for five or six days, and if any problems developed I should call him.

This was a simple, routine request—nothing more—yet it profoundly inflated my narcissistic ego. Praise was, indeed, the elixir of my life. Two days later, however, my rush was abruptly quashed.

I was seated at the boss's desk, busy dictating, when I heard someone exhale. I looked up. Sal was leaning against the door jamb—silent. He had a cigarette in his mouth which was rare for him. I sensed something awful, but managed to put on a smile, and tried to sound upbeat as I greeted him, "Hey! You're back early. What's up?"

He ignored my question, and instead got right to the point. "You know Roger Evans?"

"Sure. I trained under him," I admitted. I didn't add we'd become arch enemies and he'd succeeded in blacklisting me in Houston. "Why?"

"Well, for starters, he doesn't think too much of you."

All of a sudden the room was hot as hell. "Whaddaya mean?"

"I went to a lecture he gave yesterday morning on scoliosis, and later that afternoon while I was walking around the exhibit hall, I happened to see him by the Zimmer booth. I knew you had trained in Houston where he practices, so I went up to him, introduced myself, and asked if he remembered you. His exact words were, 'Scheiner . . . Jim Scheiner? Yeah, I remember him. Jewish kid, right?'

I then asked him how you were as a resident. I couldn't believe it when he said you were, 'one of the worst residents we ever had.' I asked him why and he said you were an 'unethical, piss-poor, hot dog of a surgeon.' Before he walked off, he said, 'If I were you, I'd be careful of that hot-shot.' He scared the shit out of me. That's why I'm back."

"For God's sake, Sal, I was just a resident, a fuckin' student. He's so wrong about me. I'm a good doctor and a good surgeon. You know it and he knows it."

As I looked at him, I could tell he wasn't buying. He was not only upset, he was scared stiff. He was wondering who the hell I was and what the hell my intentions were. I knew he believed what that anti-Semite Evans had said to him and was kicking himself for having taken me in. Now, he would always have to be on guard. He was trapped. Unfortunately, because of our contract, he couldn't get rid of me, at least not for a year.

"Go on home," he spat with a flick of his wrist. "We'll talk about it later."

I knew he was hoping, when I got home, I would pack my bags and never return. I should have, but I needed the job.

Under the circumstances, any well-adjusted individual would have reacted with a reasonable amount of fear and anxiety. Evans' censure and its consequences, however, were as traumatic and violating to my ego as a high-velocity gunshot wound. I was crushed with humiliation and the sense of extreme failure. I needed praise and admiration, not abuse. I needed to be perceived as someone special, not as an incompetent fool. My life felt meaningless and empty.

Languishing in despair, I dragged myself, head-down, toward the back door where my car was parked. The doors of the examining rooms were open since it was too early for patients. As I shuffled by the one nearest the back, my eye caught the glint of the steel, medication tray sitting on the cabinet beside the examining table. I slithered into the room. Hearing nothing, I quickly looked up and down the hall and then, with my hands shaking, snatched a handful of syringes and the squat, heavy-glass vial of Demerol. I jammed all of it into my pants pocket, and calmly walked out into the cool, crisp morning.

I drove around aimlessly, both the Chieftain and my gray matter on automatic. It must have been hours before I found myself parked in a vacant spot, brooding over what had transpired, and what I should do. I longed to unburden my mind by talking it over with Hannah, but I couldn't. I knew that any emotional stress could cause her to go into labor, and since she was only 28 weeks, she could lose the twins. I had to keep silent.

I thought of the soothing comfort bulging my pocket and how quickly the crystal-clear vial of liquid ecstasy could put an end to my torment. I took it out and studied it. Suddenly, my entire body began to tingle and quiver with anticipation, and within seconds, I was on the edge of a maddening craving. I tried to suppress it. But this arousal, this perverse titillation, suddenly exploded into a tempest with such fury, I had no choice . . .

I plucked out a "hypo" from my pocket, frantically tore open its wrapping, and pushed the needle of it through the rubber stopper and into the clear liquid within the vial warming in the palms of my sweaty, palsied hands. I withdrew three cc's, held the needle high, pushed the plunger in to eject the residual air—along with a drop or two of the precious liquid—savagely thrust it right though my pants, and "banged it" deep within the muscular core of my thigh. With a fleeting gleam of guilt I pulled it out, slouched back against the seat, and closed my eyes to await the warm, orgasmic shudder.

It was shadowing and silent when I awoke, feeling as if I were adrift somewhere in a sea of confusion until a distant bark roused me back to reality and the thought of Hannah.

When I got to our apartment, it was dark and hushed. I dashed around like a crackbrain flicking every light switch and screaming, "Hannah, Hannah . . ." No one was there.

Terrified, I ran into the kitchen to call someone. But who? The police? As I stood there trying to pull myself together, I saw a note in Hannah's handwriting in the middle of the kitchen table by a pepper shaker:

J –

6:20 p.m.

Couldn't find you!

Water broke!

Went to Columbia Hospital.

Hurry!

H

HANNAH

The day the twins were born, they had isolated Hannah as much as they possibly could in a relatively quiet corner, away from the constant traffic and the often-frenetic goings-on that complement the care of critical patients. She was lying flat on her back, looking both brave and frightened. I leaned over the side rails, kissed her lovingly, then solemnly stood at the side of the bed holding her hand.

Within a few minutes, two OR nurses, chattering gaily and gushing with optimism, arrived pushing a clattering gurney. I helped them lift Hannah onto it and continued to hold her hand as they carefully pushed the stretcher to the delivery room. I dragged myself down to the hospital cafeteria thinking the coffee might be better if I paid for it. It wasn't. I drank it there, and then bought another to take back to the lounge. Two anxious hours passed before the door opened and her doctor told me, "Everybody's fine, Jim."

I was beside myself with joy. Hannah and I had created two healthy twin boys. We were the parents of three sons. We were a *family*. For the first time in years, I wanted to talk to my parents, let them know what was going on in my life. After brief visits to the nursery and my drained wife, I drove home and picked up the phone. I couldn't believe I actually remembered the number. But as I dialed, I suddenly found myself overwhelmed by panic. I couldn't do it. With a violently shaking hand I put the receiver down. Twenty minutes later, I was rejoicing again. My pal Demerol had seen to that.

ANTOINE'S REVENGE

Silence and solitude are rare commodities in prison. I found their absence to be maddening. It wasn't just the loud chatter, joking, and cursing going on at all hours that caused my ire; it was the profusion of screaming, shrieking, noise generators which expanded and delineated their owner's "space"—the boom boxes—that made me crazy. They were on round-the-clock, everywhere, their powerful speakers blasting a continual clamor of crude, repulsive, meaningless rap. To me, the "new fish" at the mansion who some black cons liked to call honky, marshmallow, pink, snake, whitey, and for some reason, monkey, this freakish, avant-garde, black craze was unbearable.

Late one night, I couldn't take it anymore. I lost it. I was in the library, needing to be alone, wanting to read.

It must have been after one in the morning, and although I was trying to focus on Steinbeck's <u>Tortilla Flat</u>—I heard the click of the door behind me being unlatched and, a moment later, violently thrown open. Jolted back to reality, I turned around in my chair and almost fell out of it at the sight of my nemesis, Antoine Dubois, standing in the doorway leaning on his cane, sneering at me.

He was holding a boom box in his right hand. As I watched, stunned and in silence, he approached the table where I had settled, and gently placed it exactly in its center. Then he reached over my shoulder with a spider-like arm, and with an over-long thumb and index finger turned it on, causing it to erupt into a blasting rap that reverberated throughout the room. He then hobbled to the other side of the table and glared at me, daring me to react. It was as if he had thrown down a gauntlet.

I just stared back at him, hanging tough, waiting for his next move. To my immense relief, he finally struck the floor sharply with his cane and limped out of the room, abandoning his ghetto blaster.

I stood up and began to walk the floor, trying to comprehend what the hell was going on, but more importantly, what I should do. One thing I knew for certain though was that I and I alone was going to have to deal with this situation.

As I paced round and round, I could feel my adrenaline rise. Soon this omnipotent biochemical was my boiling blood. Every one of my senses, my rage, and my strength were magnified and intensified a hundred-fold, making me invincible, or so I thought. In truth, I was out of control. I glared at that satanic box with loathing and contempt. Then, I took it in both hands, lifted it above my head, and with a single, swift motion hurled it against the wall and silenced it. Forever.

The abrupt silence was soothing but short-lived. Just as I settled down again with my feet propped on the table top, ready to resume reading Steinbeck, Antoine returned and hurled himself at me screaming, "Yo motha-fuckin, hooknose, cunt. I'll kill yo white ass!" It was his turn to be out of control.

Shielding my face with my hands, I tried to stand up, but I slipped and fell, striking the top of my head on one of the legs of the table. Blood quickly blurred my vision. I was confused, in turmoil, clearly outmatched.

I was unable to elude or defend myself against the relentless pounding of Antoine's fists and cane. Just before losing consciousness, I caught sight of a crude knife made from a toothbrush handle and a razorblade in Antoine's raised left hand. As he was about to slash me, I heard Bobby's soft, familiar voice implore, "Drop the steel, buckwheat." And then, nothingness.

RECIDIVISM

All the Demerol in Ianerella's office was now kept in a locked drawer. The vial I took when Ianerella had returned abruptly from New Orleans was found missing by none other than Trudy, the receptionist. When she confronted me about it, I told her a patient had probably stolen it, and that Dr. Ianerella should have known better than to have narcotics lying around in plain sight. I knew she didn't buy my story, but there was no way she could prove I took it.

I needed drugs, badly. I had just been slapped with a shocking summons in a major malpractice suit. All I'd done was refer a middle-aged woman with a slipped disc to a neurosurgeon who, while removing the disc, tore into a major artery leaving her crippled. Had a vascular surgeon not been close by she would have hemorrhaged to death. I knew I wasn't to blame, but the stress of it all was getting to me.

I thought of writing a phony script for myself, but was afraid to do so. Then I thought of calling a drug rep and getting some samples of Percodan or Dilaudid, but again I was afraid, knowing Trudy was watching me closely.

Halfway home, I again considered writing a phony script, but still in control, I thought better of it. I tried to contain my craving as long as I could, but it only got worse. I started to shake and began to panic. I had to have it!

A few blocks from our apartment, I pulled in to the Walgreens' lot. While parked under a dulled, yellow street lamp, I wrote a script for 12, 50 mg. tablets of Demerol, hoping the small number of pills would reduce any suspicion that the prescription was a fraud. I made it out to one of my patients, Daniel Robinson. After signing my name, scared to death by what I was doing, I crumpled it. Two minutes later, I wrote another, got out of the car, walked to the back of the store, and handed it to the pharmacy clerk.

The clerk informed me that it would be at least an hour before the prescription was ready, which was just about closing time. I thanked her, walked out, and drove home scared as hell, knowing that what I had done was wrong, so very wrong. I stood the chance of losing everything I had practically killed myself for, even going to jail, but it just didn't seem to matter. I had to have it. I couldn't overcome the formidable power and persuasiveness of my grievous, damnable need.

When I got home, I lied to Hannah, telling her I'd forgotten to buy cigarettes and had gone back out again.

"I'll be right back," I told her.

"Get me a pack, too," she called out from the kitchen.

Driving back to Walgreens, I kept whispering to myself, *The cops, they're waiting for me. I know it, but I gotta have it. Demerol is the only thing that can help me.* I was out of control. I had to take the chance. The craving was relentless. I had to get that shit. I had to! And I had to get it now! The damned store was about to close!

I walked in just as the lights were dimming on and off. There were two or three customers standing around the pharmacy, waiting. Thank God, no one knew me. I asked the clerk if Mr. Robinson's prescription was ready. She said she would check with the pharmacist. When she returned, she said, "He'll get to it in just a minute."

Then I thought, *They're tripping the alarm to the police station, and now they're stalling for time. I'm trapped!* I looked at the pill merchant who was counting out a bottle of gray and pink capsules: Darvocet. In the midst of his counting, he abruptly stopped and looked straight at me, at first frowning, then smiling. I turned away and started looking for a TV camera. I was sure they were videotaping me. I instinctively put my hand over my face.

The lights were dimmer now, and someone announced the store was closing. When I looked up, I was alone. I wanted to get out of there, but I knew it was too late.

"Mister Robinson. Mister Robinson! MISTER ROBINSON!"

It didn't dawn on me that the clerk was calling the name I had written on the prescription, until she came out from behind the counter.

"Your prescription is ready. You can pay for it here."

The parking lot was empty except for my car.

Emotionally exhausted from the ordeal, I sat in a stupor staring out the side window of the car. Then, with trembling fingers, I tore open the small, white, paper bag and removed its contents: a white-capped, brown cylinder labeled with some sort of warning directive that I couldn't make out in the semi-dark. Pressing down hard on the cap and then twisting, it came off. I tilted out three, small, white tablets in my palm, bent over, hacked up some phlegm, put the malicious magic in my mouth, raised up, swallowed, and closed my eyes. Ten minutes later the drug kicked in, slowly winging me to another existence: this one, however, not a reality, but rather a fools' paradise.

As I drove home, steadily mellowing out all of my cares—the unjustified blacklisting, the impending malpractice suit, and Ianarella's loss of faith in me—soon evaporated. By the time I entered the apartment, I was in the dead-center of a transcendent euphoria. Yes, the big "D"—so easy, so effective, so divine, so cruel.

ANTOINE'S REVENGE

"Can you hear me? Open your eyes. Hi, Mr. Scheiner. My name is Brian. I'm your nurse. You're in the Recovery Room. Your surgery's over. You're waking up."

"Surgery?! What the hell happened?" I managed a hoarse whisper.

"One of your friends over at the prison got pretty mad and really messed you over. You were in a coma when you got here, but the CT of your brain was OK. You were also bleeding from your stomach and from a horrible laceration on your head. The doctor, thank God, was able to stop the bleeding by putting a tube down your stomach. When he gets here he'll explain everything. Try not to worry, you'll be all right."

After checking my pulse and a quick but discerning glance at my cardiac rhythm flitting across the monitor on the wall, he gazed down at me, shook his head, and frowned for a minute or so, seemingly perplexed and lost in thought. Then for some reason, he squeezed my hand and murmured; "I can't locate your wife. No one answered the phone. I'll keep trying."

The cool weight of a stethoscope and the escalating squeeze of a blood-pressure cuff ballooning around my arm woke me after a short sleep. I watched, half asleep, as Brian pressed down on the diaphragm of his 'scope, and, while listening, slowly released the pressure in the cuff. When he was done, he looked at me and said he still hadn't been able to get a hold of Hannah. I asked him to please keep trying.

Four days later, I left the hospital, anemic, depressed, and very much afraid. I begged to stay on a few more days, but the Federal

Bureau of Prisons, which was footing the "medicals," maintained there was no reason I couldn't convalesce in one of their beds under the supervision of their "very competent and very experienced medical staff." Besides, I was a convicted felon.

Back home at the mansion, I slept for two weeks, never once being seen by any of the very competent, very experienced medical staff. Then early one morning, I opened my eyes and saw the administrator bent over me.

"I just came to tell ya," he said, very kindly, "R&R's over. This ain't the Hilton, ya know. Toilets need cleanin', boy." Then he added, "I don't think you'll have any more trouble, seein' as you said, you don't know which of your schoolmates tried to kill ya."

But he knew that I knew who it was, and I knew he understood why I had to keep silent.

MALPRACTICE

It was two years, almost to the day, after her botched surgery, that her lawyer successfully convinced the jury that Mrs. Emily Simmons had been a victim of a "flagrant and grievous act of malpractice" and that, legally, the neurosurgeon and I had been engaged in a joint enterprise as regards Mrs. Simmons' care. They felt, after only four hours of deliberation, that my colleague owed her $1.5 million in damages for his wrongful act. I, for having the reckless indiscretion of referring this patient to him, owed her $250,000 which, fortunately, was covered by insurance. The day the verdict and judgment were announced, contrary to reason, I was as unfazed and as calm as could be. My Demerol saw to that.

Two months after she became well-to-do from the malpractice settlement, Mrs. Simmons died of hepatocellular carcinoma, a known complication of cirrhosis.

Being sued for malpractice, dragged into court, and put on trial proved to be one of the most burdensome and pervasive experiences of my professional life. In my clearer moments, I couldn't believe I was held liable for the conduct and actions of another doctor. Even though I was nowhere near the OR when that neurosurgeon tore that hole in Simmons' artery, in the eyes of the law, I was just as responsible. I was made to feel as if I had gone out and hired that bastard to complicate her life. I felt helpless, a pawn of the legal system.

I was angry and I hated everyone—the whole fuckin' world—for what they were doing to me. But above all, it was a terrifying, scathing denunciation of what I thought of myself, and worst of all, what others might think of me. I was sure that any perception of me as a person of importance and competence would be shattered.

The legal proceedings, as they all are, were lengthy and devastating. There seemed to be no end to the meetings, interrogatories, depositions, and questions. It was an incessant thorn, pricking me day and night, and often waking me from a deep sleep. It debilitated me, emotionally and physically.

Only Demerol helped me get through this, so I made sure I had a steady supply. After that first unnerving visit to Walgreens pharmacy, writing fake scripts became routine for me. I would rotate them around at least ten different pharmacies to avoid suspicion, and usually telephone them in, so as not to have to wait and become identifiable.

BOBBY

His flinty face and his wiry body were at odds with a soul that had gotten soft with sorrow and misery. He had been the "Master" of the toilets for over five years and was due to be sprung in three or four weeks. I was his replacement. He was my teacher.

"Lot's o' bad folk here, Jew boy, like your friend, Antoine. Better pray he don' come after you again."

So everyone knew. Of course they did. What the hell did I think I was in: a Boy Scout camp? There are no secrets here.

"You think he might?" I spit out sourly.

"For a fact, 'less you learns how to handle yourself an' I'm not talking 'bout carrying violence in your back pocket."

"Whaddaya mean?"

"See, Jew boy," he spelled out in a voice tinged with bitter resignation, "to cut it here you gots ta get respect, and it don' necessarily take trashin' or carvin' someone up to get it. You just gots ta learn to stand up for yourself—hang tough. You just gotta be strong in the head. You gotta stan' your ground."

As he shuffled away, he cautioned over his shoulder, "Be careful, boy. Mind you own business, show some respect, and don' ever, ever trust anyone. An' o' yeah, remember, snitches get stitches."

And, oh, yeah, I recalled, *you can steal, but you never squeal.*

As I continued to scrub the toilets and the bathroom floor on my hands and knees, I couldn't get the image of Antoine and the incident in the library out of my mind. *Why was he angry enough to kill me?* I pushed the rough brush over the tiles vengefully. *What did he have against me?*

My mind went in circles, the way my hand was directing the scrub brush, the way Leonard had taught me. Did everyone clean their floors this way, I wondered? My mother never scrubbed floors; that would have been beneath her. Hannah had a housekeeper; I'd never watched her do housework.

Then my mind circled back to Antoine's gunshot wound that hot night in Houston . . . My glib, racist remark . . . The look on his face . . . The way fate brought us together again here in this prison . . . *Prison, bah, the great equalizer!* . . . His boom-box, delineating his sacred space . . . His challenging me . . . His pent-up, justifiable rage . . .

The next time I ran into Bobby, outside on the grounds on a sunny day, I thanked him for saving my life and offered him my hand. He shook it and smiled.

"Bobby, I need to know: Why do you think Antoine tried to kill me?"

"You really wanna know? Well, the short, one-word answer to your question is: racism. In more than one way, you and your kind have crippled Antoine Dubois for life.

"Racists are guilty of actions designed to block the advancement of a people. You bad-mouth us, you knock us down, and then you shit on us. You look down on us as second-rate nobodies, garbage. That, my dear white brother, is pure and simple racism."

Bobby seemed to know, intuitively, exactly who and what I was— an arrogant, close-minded bigot. And he was aware, even more than I, of the snobbish, apartheid deeply rooted in every level of American society. He and I talked for the better part of the afternoon. With his words, he drew me into his world: a dark, frightening, tragic world of desperation and despair. More importantly, he made me feel ashamed, since what he said was justified and true.

In the seemingly endless days that followed, I took advantage of every chance I got to meet and talk with Bobby. For the first time, it seemed, I truly listened to another human being when he spoke about his life. And he, in turn, appeared to care about mine.

VERNON

The phony good-byes and synthetic well-wishes over, I drove away from Sal Ianarella's clinic mournful that our relationship had been besieged by rude awakenings and lost illusions and anxious because I was now on my own.

I had taken out a lease on some cheap, office space in the basement of an old, three-storied building around the corner from the Good Samaritan Hospital. Needing a girl-Friday, I called up Kelly Services, and hired the first young woman they sent over, a naïve 19-year-old named Elaine, with suspect secretarial skills.

Unable to afford a nurse, I hired a young man with a leg crippled from polio who had been an orderly at the "Good Sam." Vernon was so happy to free himself of the servile chores and disrespect he'd known as an orderly, he jumped at my offer. And when I suggested twice the salary he had been getting, and a promise to throw my old car into the deal whenever I could afford a new one, he leaped into my arms and kissed me.

Within six months that musty office was humming. The three of us were busy, and the money was starting to flow: enough to put a down payment on a cozy, little split-level house for Hannah and me and the kids, and give Elaine and Vern well-deserved raises. And, in no time, Vern got the old station wagon, and I got *the* car: a purring, emerald-green, Cadillac Eldorado—my "Jew-canoe."

By then, Vern had become indispensable, even taking histories and performing preliminary physical exams. He almost always stayed late and frequently worked Saturdays, but at least once or twice a month—just a bit too often—he would call in sick.

I knew he drank. On occasion he showed up hung-over, smelling of whiskey, unshaven, disheveled, and his limp more evident than usual. I spoke to him on several occasions. I urged him to try to control his drinking. But he would still call in sick. I knew he needed alcohol the way I needed Demerol. I could relate.

Then I hit upon a solution to Vern's drinking. It came to me one evening when the A.H. Robins pharmaceutical rep was sitting in my office detailing their muscle relaxant. Before leaving—besides the usual freebies, such as pens and pads —he left samples of Robins' premier pain med, Pheraphen #3: large, green and black capsules filled with acetaminophen and codeine which, although not as potent as Demerol, are nonetheless, highly addictive. The samples were in bottles of 100's which I was thinking of using myself, in lieu of Demerol, since they were so easy to come by. I was sitting staring at the sample bottles when the "surrogate solution" came to me.

Knowing that Methadone was being prescribed as a less dangerous substitute for many of the hard drugs addicts favored, I thought, *Why not something to take the place of Vern's booze? Why not try Pheraphen #3?*

It worked. Vern threw away *his* bottle, never again missed a day, and all his patients began to comment on his inspiring, irrepressible personality.

Vern was so involved with his own shtick, taking x-rays and PT, that he had trouble finding time to assist me, and Elaine was so busy with appointments, billing, scheduling surgery, and reams of typing that it was hard for her to tear herself away to chaperon examinations of female patients. One morning, both of them joined forces to inform me that if I didn't get a real nurse to help me, they were history. As luck would have it, before I even got around to advertising for a nurse, Maggie walked into my life.

BOBBY

Cleaning the five filthy commodes, the open four-headed shower, the piss-puddled trench, and the six-fauceted sink with the splintered mirror hanging above it took the better part of the morning.

It was a drudge that at first made me feel as if I were being eaten alive by a pack of rats. But I was learning patience; and under Leonard's tutelage, I was beginning to master the various disciplines—sweeping, scouring, scrubbing, swabbing, scraping, and sanitizing—like a pro. As a hot-shot surgeon I could earn $5,000 a day. This job paid 16¢ an hour.

But as hard as I slaved—"to do it right, boy, ya gots ta git down and crawl aroun', jest like a nigger"—and as neat and as fresh as I got it to look, it almost always smelled like a decomposing skunk.

After a while, however, during the solitude and simplicity of these chores, while crawling on my hands and knees like a postulant confessing, I came to know an undeniable peace and a sense of freedom. It was as if, while scrubbing out the muck of that toilet, I was scrubbing out the muck that cluttered my soul.

After a morning of cleaning, there was lunch in the mess hall, which was located in the mansion's basement, just down the hall from the library. It was euphemistically known as the "grease trough." The food, a monotonous mélange of unimaginative, tasteless glop, slop, and goop, was served cafeteria style.

Once or twice a week, for no apparent reason, the trough remained open for an hour after lunch for those who cared to tell tales and to make the best of another cup or two of coffee. Regardless, Bobby and

I were usually the only ones with stomachs stubborn enough to take advantage of it. On one such afternoon, during an explosive thunderstorm, I learned that his revolutionary spirit was forged as a child by an episode of pure evil.

From time to time, as he sketched its ugly particulars, he would stop talking and just sit staring and frowning at the intricate grid of rusting, peeling pipes across the ceiling, shaking his head slowly from side to side.

"I was born in 1942, in Valdosta, Georgia, 20 miles north of the Florida border. Like all my people in the 'gulag' in the South, I grew up bleeding a lot, sweating a lot, and crying a lot: the afterbirth of the insults, humiliations, and mistrust of the white racists who looked on all us niggers as dumb, lazy, potential criminals, and a blame for everything. If there was a hurricane, it was the niggers' fault. If there was a drought, if there was a murder, a rape, a robbery, an epidemic, anything, you name it, it was our fault.

"I was born at home, delivered by a Haitian 'granny-woman;' a part-time midwife and a part-time voodooist said to have real juju. In fact, my mama told me that when I was born, the voodooist divined that, someday, I would 'beat the white devils.' Well, looks like so far, they's beatin' me.

"I was born 74 years after the passage of the Fourteenth Amendment, which gave black citizenship and granted equal protection under the law. But, here it was 1942, and we were still only citizens in name. Hell, most of us couldn't even vote 'cause we couldn't pass the tests you had to take to qualify. It was sad, 'cause hardly anyone ever got the opportunity to learn to read or write. It wasn't until the Voting Rights Act of 1965—1965!—can you believe that? when such obstacles to voting were removed.

"When I was six, the nightriders came to the house. The Klan. It was, maybe, two in the morning, and my mama, smelling smoke, woke up lookin' at the flickering shadows of a burning cross playing on the walls of our miserable, leaky, drafty shack that sat at the edge of a wood near the cotton gin where my daddy worked. She gently woke us up, and, after shushing us, bolted the door. I remember us creeping over to the window and peeking out to see what the hell was goin' on. Because of the fire and a full moon, we could plainly see a bunch o' hooded Kluckers sittin' on horses in a circle 'round the entire shack. They all carried torches, and were armed with shotguns, rifles, or machetes, and one was playing with a heavy, coiled-up rope like a cowboy.

"A few of 'em had gotten off their horses, and were standing around that damned, flaming cross that looked to be 50 feet high, and because of the wind was really flamin' and shootin' off sparks. And, all of 'em, all of them 'mutha-fuckers' were waiting, just waiting.

"They were all silent and looked to be calm, but we all knew they were in a frenzy: freaked-out and we knew they were there because Daddy had witnessed the 'cotton-boss' brutally rape my 12-year-old cousin, Sharleen, behind a pile of cotton bales, and had testified against him in court. It was hard to believe, but that 'buckra' was found guilty by an all-white jury, and sentenced to do a 'double-sawbuck,' 20 years, on a chain gang. That pussy-bandit's name was Daryl Forrest, who just happened to be the only son of the Georgia den's Grand Dragon. Yes, Daddy knew they were comin'. He knew, for sure.

"We waited inside, and they waited outside. And then after, maybe, 15 of the longest, most dreadful minutes we ever spent, we heard a thundering voice, like someone shouting into a megaphone. 'All you mud people, get out of the house, or we'll burn it down! You niggers got one minute!'

"We were frantic. They were all over the place. There was no escaping, not for my folks, anyhow, but they saved me.

"Well, the shack was propped up on cinder blocks to keep out rattlesnakes and possums, and one of the floor planks happened to be loose. My daddy pried it open, and pushed me through, down into the darkness of that slimy, crawl space. Damned if it wasn't crawlin' with slugs and bugs and God knows what else. I'll never forget his last words to me, 'don' be afraid, son' and 'don' yo' make a sound, yo' hea', and, no matte' what; don yo' come out. Promise me, son!'"

"Just as he pushed the plank back in place, all hell broke loose. The Kluckers broke down the door, stormed into the shack, and hauled my parents outside. I crawled through the muck to the edge of the shack to see what was going on. They were tying my daddy to a tree, and when they were done, the Grand Dragon, the one with the fancy emblems on his robe just walked up to him, and after spitting in his face, shoved the butt of his gun into his mouth. I could hear the bone crush, and saw my daddy spit out at least a cup o' blood, along with teeth and pieces of bone. It made me vomit. The Grand Dragon then yelled in his face, 'We don't cotton to dirty, nigger liars, Boy!'

"They just watched him struggle for a while, and then another Klucker walked up to him, spit in his face, and shoved the butt of his gun right into my daddy's crotch causing him to, thank God, pass out because then, the ones with the machetes grabbed my mama and marched her not three feet from Daddy. They held her up, and made her watch as they hacked him to pieces. One of them, after cutting off his head, stuck it in his machete and flung it towards the shack. It rolled right next to me! It was so close I could smell the blood. But those bastards weren't done yet. They tied Mama's arms behind her back, and then threw her down on her stomach, tied her ankles together, and then bent her knees up, so they could tie her ankles to her wrists. When she was trussed like a chicken, they looped a rope over a branch of the tree they had butchered my daddy on, and tied one end to the ropes binding my mama, and hoisted her up about ten feet off the ground. While she dangled, those animals prodded her with their guns and machetes, causing her to spin like a top. Then they ripped off her nightclothes. When they were tired of 'playing' with her, they took some of the logs stacked beside the shack, built a fire under her, and slowly roasted her.

"And you know what, during all that, she never screamed, and never cried. All she did was repeat over and over, 'The Lord is my shepherd, I shall not want. . .' over and over. After a half-hour or so when the fire started to die, they added more wood, and when it was really roaring, the Grand Dragon rode his horse up to her, and with the bayonet on his rifle, slit open her belly allowing the child she was carrying to slip out. For a while, he just hung there and twirled, but then, the twisted cord separated, and he fell into the flames.

"Then the rope burnt through, causing my mama to drop into the burning embers with a thud that created a mountainous cloud of sparks and ashes, the smell of which the wind carried to where I was hiding, and made me vomit again. After she fell, they threw the chunks of meat that had been my daddy to burn along with her. And then, they rode off into the night, laughing and shouting, 'three less coons, three less baboons.'"

Bobby was drained after having exposed his wounds as was I upon hearing of them. I wanted to say something, but there was nothing I could think of to say. As a doctor, I had learned how to comfort the sick and the dying, but there was nothing I, nor anyone, could say that would, even in the slightest, give comfort or relief to such anguish.

We sat for a while, slowly sipping the last few drops of cold, bitter coffee. The room was empty, except for us, and two grubby-looking white cons quietly cleaning the tables and mopping up the floor. We could hear the ticking of the clock, whose face indicated it was just about time for the klaxon to signal the count.

MAGGIE

It was late, and everyone had gone. I had my keys out and was locking up the office when the phone rang.

A soft, sugar-coated southern drawl cooed, "Hey, y'all! This is Maggie, Dr. Pendleton's nurse? The doctah's outatown at a meetin', and I was hopin' y'all might be able to see a little boy with a hurt arm."

Rather reluctantly, I agreed to wait. And then, after an hour and a half, she made her dramatic entrance. I had seen many nurses in crisp, white uniforms but none as stunning and shapely as this one.

"Hi, Doctah! Ah'm Maggie, and this heah's Freddy! Shor doo thank-ya fer seein' us! His daddy said to do whatevah. He'll be along soon."

Maggie made herself right at home. She helped take the x-ray, develop it, and then—breathing heavily and sighing, her right breast pressed firmly against my left shoulder as we studied the view box—she pointed out with a dainty finger the fracture, a simple, greenstick break—that didn't need setting—in one of the bones just above his wrist. Maggie held him as I slapped a cast on his pudgy arm.

Afterwards, seeing the light on the percolator, she poured two cups, found a Pepsi in the fridge for Freddy, and after asking permission, lit up a filter. I then gave Freddy a Superman comic, and we sat down in my office waiting for his daddy.

While we chatted, she mentioned she was a graduate of Mississippi University School of Nursing in Jackson, and while there, had married an evangelist who, at the time, was one of the chaplains at the Obadiah Holmes Baptist Hospital where she was doing her "ob-gyn." They had two "dahlin" children.

After Freddy's father arrived, Maggie, without so much as a word, walked over to Elaine's desk, sat down, typed up a chart, found the patient info and insurance forms, and handed them to him to fill out. When he finished, she put Freddy's name in the appointment book, and instructed him and his son as to exactly what to do, and what to watch for over the next few days. I just stood there with my arms crossed—duly impressed.

When Freddy and his father had gone, Maggie looked up at me with a strange, undefinable smile on her slightly open lips. I knew she was struggling with something. When at last she opened her mouth, the cutesy, "suthen" accent was gone, replaced altogether by a voluptuous, deep-throated, straight-forward statement in the shape of a question: "You do drugs, don't you?"

She didn't need to wait for an answer. She knew. And, knowing her powers, she added in a throaty whisper, "Why don't you follow me over to my office, I have something I know you'll like." By then, I was so spellbound and possessed by her voodoo I would have followed her anywhere.

Dr. Pendleton's office was dark, but she left the lights off as she led me to his private office.

"Wait here. I'll be right back," she breathed.

She returned after a few minutes holding a syringe and needle in her right hand, and a blanket, neatly folded and draped, over her left arm. Before entering the office, she posed for a moment in the night-glow just outside the door. She was naked.

Shivering in her nakedness, but purring like a kitten, she whispered in my ear to take off my clothes. She then covered the narrow, Naugahyde examining table with the blanket.

"Lie down."

After giving two weeks' notice to Pendleton, Maggie became my nurse.

⟊

At first, with an oral slug of Demerol every few hours during the day, and an occasional fix in the evening, I was able to function. I saw patients, attended meetings, covered the ER, and operated without anyone becoming suspicious of my addiction.

Soon, however, my hunger for the more exquisite and swift sensations the injections triggered, became overpowering. I tried to hold out but soon began to yield to the needle. In a small, locked, storage room down the hall from my office, I began shooting up during the lunch break. And there, on the floor or standing, Maggie and I would often enjoy a "matinee."

Predictably, within a short time I found myself wanting it more often and more of it at a time. It didn't take long before I was pumping myself full of junk every five or six hours, 24/7. The pills had become obsolete. At home, during the night, I would get out of bed, take out the bottom drawer of the bathroom vanity, reach back for the cache of Demerol and paraphernalia hidden there, and "needle" myself. Now, I was no longer in control. I wasn't even aware that with the drug, I was barely functioning. I only knew that without it, I couldn't function at all.

I don't know how she did it, but as far as I knew, Maggie never took more than a single shot a day. She was obviously much stronger and disciplined than I. And Vern, well, he was quite content with his Pheraphens.

I knew I was taking way too much, but I couldn't help it, and Maggie just let it ride. We acted as if our perverse existence was the most natural thing in the world. Neither she nor I were the slightest bit concerned that that dammed drug had unconditionally taken over my body and my soul. The craving had become so compelling, so fierce, and so merciless that I could do nothing but surrender to it. It possessed me so completely that it smothered my conscience. I never even thought of what I was doing to myself, my patients, or my family. Nothing entered my mind but the need to get high.

I kept taking more and more. Then one night I told Maggie to shoot it in my veins. She was hesitant, saying it was too dangerous, and I really needed to cut down. I didn't want to hear that. I didn't want to hear anything. I just wanted the drug in my veins. For the first time, since we had become a drug duet, I could see she was scared. Yet, she acquiesced.

It only took a few days before I had ceased to mainline for the ecstasy of it. From then on, I was doing it solely to keep from getting sick: from feeling the craving that made itself felt every single time I started to come down, which was precisely five hours after the last "bang." Then, if another bang wasn't right there, I would become enraged, panicky, terrified, because I knew I would soon become debilitatingly sick if I didn't immediately quash the craving.

AN UNCOMPROMISING AGENDA

I f you want breakfast, you grunt out of a gnarly mattress at precisely 4 a.m. when the entire place suddenly erupts with light. Heavy-eyed, you pray no one has stolen the shoes you forgot to stow in your locker. If not, you still grumble because you're saying to yourself, *Dammit, it's pitch black outside and who the fuck feels like getting dressed and trudging downstairs to eat that piss and punk. But, shit, I'm starving.*

Then at 4:30 a.m., when that fiendish whistle shrieks and you're waiting, leaning with your head against the bed post, for the first of the day's body counts, you really start to grumble—aloud now. And you start breathing hard and shaking your head because you're still hemorrhaging inside, thinking about how you, the big-shot orthopedic surgeon, ended up in this human ware house whose stench will never clear out of your nostrils.

The pain-in-the-ass count over, you desperately need to pee, and if someone hasn't stolen your toothpaste or brush, you slog, with eyes closed, the 63 footsteps to the toilet, the 24 more to the 16-step stairwell, and then 38 to the cafeteria, where you sit at 5 a.m. sipping from a cup of sugared misery. You peck lifelessly at a plate of slop that is destined to lie like an aching lump in your stomach until nudged out by the slop you eat at lunch.

Not in any hurry, you have a second cup of what they call coffee. At least it's hot. And then you trudge up to the toilets to work.

One often hears that prison camp is more like a country club than a penitentiary. Those who have done time there, though, will quickly disabuse you of this fallacy. "How in hell," they might say, "can it be, when every fuckin' morning, while you're trying to shake off nightmares, a runaway freight train loaded with despair plows right into you?" And there is no one there to help you because no one cares.

No, Petersburg is no country club. It's a purgatory with a revolving door called recidivism, oiled by a system determined to destroy the things that define one as a human being. There are no tutors to teach anyone a way of life better than the one that got us here. There are no doctors to heal moral diseases or to suture the remnants of shattered souls. There are only correctional officers—a.k.a. screws, hacks, roaches, bullies, goons, and worse names—who don't give a shit.

Inasmuch as doing society's dirty work is a dangerous, thankless, low-paying job, you can imagine the type of person this profession attracts. For all they care, we could rot. You'd think they'd at least break up a fight, a rape, or a stabbing once in a while, instead of just milling around and talking as if they were the ones doing time.

All they care about is the fuckin' count. They want to find you standing quietly beside your bunk as soon as that nerve-racking whistle stops blowing. It blows six times every day at precisely the same times. Should someone be missing, God forbid, you just have to stand there, no matter how long, until the lost are found, dead or alive. Nobody cares which. What matters is that the count is correct. The count symbolizes prison: life reduced to numbers; an exact place and precise time for everything.

AN APATHETIC ZOMBIE

Getting my Demerol wasn't a problem. I had a legitimate reason for keeping a supply on hand, for treating my many patients who had fractures or dislocations who came to the office. Instead of using a patient's name for these scripts, however, it was perfectly legal to label them, "For Office Use," on the presumption the drug was to be given to patients, not the doctor or the nurse. It was all so convenient.

Just upstairs, on the lobby floor, was a small drugstore whose owner, a somewhat shady "pill peddler," had a rule of never questioning any prescription that crossed his counter. He was fond of saying, "I fill 'em, I don't write 'em." That being the case, without so much as a wink, he would fill all the scripts for injectable Demerol that Vern or Maggie brought up.

We didn't dare, however, try to get Demerol from the large, drug store chains like Walgreens or Rite-Aid. The salaried druggists who worked there were, as a rule, diligent and earnest. They were trained to keep an eye out for fraudulent prescriptions, and for those who misused or abused medication. Injectable Demerol is not the usual pain medication for the man on the street. A questionable script for it would arouse their immediate suspicion, and a prompt call to the police.

And we had another source: mail order. All we had to do was send a prescription to any one of a number of mail order houses throughout the country that sold medical supplies, including drugs. In a few days, a neatly wrapped UPS carton containing enough injectable

Demerol for an army arrived at my front door. Not only that, we got it wholesale.

༄

Injecting the liquid poison was like adding fuel to the fires of my addiction. It wasn't long before my level of functioning bordered on incompetence. The junk was thinking and acting for me. It had rendered my reasoning faculties so languid as to be, for all intents and purposes, inert. As a result, anything that required sober, serious thought and concentration was close to impossible. I had been reduced, in essence, to an apathetic zombie, and yet, I was treating and even performing major surgery on hundreds of human beings. Anyone could see I was a junkie, but no one tried to stop me.

My body soon degenerated into a dried-up, ashen-colored, corpse, complete with the sordid stigmata of the addict—scars, scabs, bloodstains, blood clots, and, of course, the telltale tracks that never led anywhere. And still, even with this display, no one stepped in.

I didn't know to care anymore. What difference did it make that I had lost so much weight that my clothes were falling off me, that the line of holes in my belt reached almost around, or that Hannah, as often as not, had to remind me to shave. What difference did it matter what the hell I looked like? No one cared, so why should I? What mattered was that I had the next dose somewhere nearby, ready to go.

༄

As long as I used Demerol in pill form, Hannah never realized I was an addict, simply because she couldn't see it in my eyes. Had she been sure, and God knows I wish she had, she would have done something—anything—to stop it. But the day she became convinced, without doubt, that I was a Janus doctor, she couldn't do anything.

It happened early one morning, just a few days after that first, mad, demented tryst with Maggie. I was in the shower drying off when Hannah abruptly opened the door and stepped in to retrieve the razor she had left in the soap dish. She was taken by surprise, not only at finding me there, but by what she saw. There were just three needle marks on the front of my thigh and they were minute. When she saw them, her eyes widened drastically, as if they were going to explode from the horror of them. She turned away, grabbed the razor, and stepped out, but not fast enough to conceal the look: a grim, condemnatory expression that would betray itself as the blood drained from her face at the dismay of what she had seen. Now, she knew.

CHESTER

L ike everything else within the confines of the mansion's walled city, the policy of apartheid was in force during meals. Just as the whites walked far behind the blacks on the track, so, too, they stood patiently at the end of the line until the brothas trays had been generously loaded. We ate on heavy steel tables onto which four hard bucket seats had been welded, giving them the appearance of school-yard whirligigs. There were 24 of these whimsical tables securely bolted to the floor, and set in five rows of four. The farthest row from the line was reserved exclusively for the white diners. The tables were, in all likelihood, made uncomfortable to speed up the meals, but that really wasn't necessary, since one doesn't tend to linger over prison cuisine.

Twice monthly, in an effort to curb unrest and rebellion, fried chicken and mashed potatoes was the *plat du jour*. You could always tell when the day came, since every brotha in that prison camp would be waiting in line at least an hour before serving time, wound-up with anticipation—rapping, laughing, and drooling.

Since second helpings were not allowed, many of the brothas would beseech the whites to sell their portions, bidding up to a dollar or a pack of smokes, or offering to trade fried chicken for future pork chops which many blacks, especially the Muslims, refused to eat.

Having sold my chicken, I'd fill up on wilting, browning lettuce; soppy, 'mushed' potatoes, the kind out of a box that actually dissolved in your mouth; hefty, yellow cobblestones, said to be cornbread; and slippery "goldfish," said to be sliced peaches, the dessert, served four out of five days: Jell-O, the other.

One afternoon as I walked out of the library, I smelled a rather rank odor surging from the direction of the mess hall. Curious as to what was on the menu, I asked the unsmiling, uniform posted at the door.

"Soul food," he mumbled without looking up. I, of course, had heard of that particular, black cuisine that had originated in the South, but, like most whites, had absolutely no idea as to its makeup. I soon, however, found out from my dining companion for that evening, Chester Carroll.

Before being gifted for good behavior and allowed to spend the final year of his sentence at the camp, Chester had spent 20 locked up in a six-by-twelve foot, reinforced-steel-barred coop in the bastille known as Leavenworth—in isolation. He said that soul food was served regularly at that notorious institution, and, as a result, and also because of his black wife, he had developed a taste for it. In fact, he had not only loved it, he considered himself an expert on what he termed, "Blackplate."

The mound of hominy grits was the only item on my tray I could identify, except for a sticky gob of black-eyed peas which, in prison vernacular, are known as jawbreakers. Chester identified a greenish-black, soggy lump as probably collard or mustard greens. And the pale-gray, tubular things, which I at first mistook for pasta, Chester said were actually the bowels of a hog, known as chitlins! I couldn't stomach that; nor could I get myself to bite into a nut-brown, slimy hunk of blubber spotted with small clusters of glistening bones and flecks of red meat, which I was told was the ankle joint or hock of a hog. I lifted it out of the tray with my fingers, since it would not admit the tines of the plastic fork, and placed it on Chester's tray, as payment for his shared culinary knowledge.

I was about to ask Chester why he always carried his Bible with him when I looked up and there was Bobby—dressed in his familiar, Panther uniform, complete with Ray-Bans—once again, daringly breaking prison protocol. He was walking, with his tray held aloft, amidst a roomful of stares, murmurs, and shaking heads towards the white element seated at the "back of the bus."

When he reached my whirligig, he politely, and somewhat complaisantly, asked if he could sit with us. I told him we would be delighted to have him join us for dinner, but Chester, not sure exactly what was going down, and, perhaps, feeling intimidated, wanted "out of there," and in his seemingly unnatural, soprano voice asked Bobby if he wanted him to leave. Our guest, however, who appeared to know Chester, gently placed a hand on his shoulder and insisted he stay, and gently blurting out, "I hear you're gonna be 'hittin' the bricks' next week, 'Chess' ol' boy. I came over here to wish you luck, and, being a busybody, had to find out what you're gonna do out there."

Chester's mouth gaped, his rosy cheeks paled, and he started blinking his eyes, furiously. "Whatever are you talking about, Bobby? No one said anything about me bein' sprung."

With a wink and a grin, Bobby sassed, "Trust me on this, ol' bean."

Like many inmates, Chester, at sometime during his long stretch had "come to Jesus." He was a born-again Christian. His wife, a black, elementary school teacher, had somehow convinced the minister of the Mount Moriah Baptist Church, where she attended services, to hire her husband as a sexton when he was released. The job entailed doing just about everything from ringing the bell to digging the graves in the small cemetery out back.

The church, ironically, was located just around the corner from the Texaco gas station where, 23 years before, Elvis Mumford found the preserved body of his son, "little" Jimmy Mumford, floating in the 100-gallon drum filled with waste oil he was illegally emptying in a nearby creek. Chester had drowned the boy in that sludge nine months earlier, after he had sodomized him.

Practically all the parents of the children attending Sunday School at Mount Moriah had become enraged upon hearing that a child molester, let alone a *white*, child molester, was to become the sexton, but when the head of the Virginia NAACP, Reverend Baraka El-Shabazz, spoke at a Sunday service and urged the congregation to, "act like Christians: forgive and give the man a chance," they relented. Besides, it had become common knowledge that "Chester the Molester," during his initiation at Leavenworth, had been gagged, forcefully dragged into a shower room, and there, on the wet floor, an inmate, using a glass shard, had crudely, but effectively, cut his balls off. "So really brethren, there is nothing to worry about now, is there? This pervert will be doing his kneeling at the altar instead of behind little boys. Do I hear an amen?!"

Having made known his immediate future, Chester bolted down the rest of his soul food, excused himself, and left, clutching his disintegrating, leather-bound Bible, swollen with countless bookmarks.

HANNAH

Hannah was sitting cross-legged and hunched over in the middle of the living room floor, her glazed eyes staring lifelessly at her hands, tightly clenched in her lap. She was practically covered in blood, even her mussed hair had become matted with grume. She was dressed in nothing but sweat socks, panties and a bra, one strap of which had slipped over her shoulder to her elbow. Both of her wrists were crudely bound in bloodied handkerchiefs, and blood was still escaping. Lourdes, our housekeeper, in a trance, was cradling and rocking Hannah in her arms. I felt Hannah's pulse in her neck. It was slow and steady, indicating that often what looks like a loss of a lot of blood, really isn't. She wasn't in shock.

I called an ambulance, and while waiting for it to arrive, Lourdes managed to tell me, between sobs, that she had found Hannah like this when she got there. She had tied handkerchiefs around her slashed wrists, just before calling me at my office. She had no idea what provoked this apparent suicide attempt. But I did.

At the ER, they immediately gave Hannah an injection of Thorazine. While the resident was sewing her up, I called our family physician, Dr. Rosenbaum. After telling him what was going on, he sighed, "I'm sorry, Jim . . . sounds like a severe, depressive episode, but since it's been a few months since the babies were born, it's probably not a postpartum thing. Do you think you'll be able to drive her down to Georgetown University Hospital? I'd like her to see a dear friend of mine, Sarah Fromm, a psychiatrist."

Dr. Fromm was alone, reading in her office, by the time we got there. She was an elderly, slight woman dressed in a long, white, lab coat. Her neat, gray pageboy framed a comely, concerned face.

She wheeled Hannah, still asleep, into an examining room, and tried to rouse her for an examination, but was unable to do so. From what I told her had transpired, however, she was sure that Hannah had lost touch with reality, and needed to be hospitalized, "You see, Doctor," she said with a German accent, "she may very well try again to take her life. She needs to be under continual observation, at least 'til we find out and treat what is troubling her."

Hannah was admitted to the psychiatric facility within the hospital. After the door closed on Hannah, Dr. Fromm asked me if I had time for a cup of tea. She said she needed to get some background information.

She questioned me briefly about Hannah's life, especially during the past month. During that time frame, I told her, Hannah *had* changed. She stopped cooking meals, just leaving TV dinners in the fridge for me; she stopped bringing in, or even reading the mail or the Post. During sex she seemed to be a thousand miles away, and I told her of having asked Hannah if there was anything wrong when, on two separate occasions, her mother called, and she had told Lourdes to tell her she was either asleep or out and would call back. As far as I knew, she hadn't.

After telling her all that I could think of, Dr. Fromm bluntly asked if *I* drank or took drugs. Like any addict, I was able to look her straight in the face and lie, but there was unmistakable doubt written all over her face. I could see that, but she let it go.

I know I should have realized Hannah was depressed. I should have tried to help her. I know I would have if she had been one of my patients. But I was oblivious, and being drugged up with Demerol and Maggie, I just didn't give a damn. Nothing else, not even my wife, not even my children, mattered. Nothing mattered . . . other than my next dose.

❦

The instant I arrived home after that meeting with Fromm, I ran straight to the bedroom bathroom, took out the bottom drawer of the vanity, got on my knees, reached back, but felt nothing but a narrow, wooden ledge. I bent down further and looked into the emptiness. Nothing. My heart stopped. My stuff was gone. Impossible! How?

Thinking, perhaps, I had hidden them behind a different drawer, I yanked another out, and then another, and then another, and then there were no more. Frantically, I reached back and looked in each opening, but again, nothing. Nothing. By then I was in a rage, sweating and trembling with fear and anger and guilt, for now I knew, for sure, that what Hannah had found here had pushed her over the edge.

Now, I really needed it. I bolted out to the car, sped over to the office, and as fast as I could, tied a tourniquet around my calf, and pumped a load of shit into a large vein—one of the few left—on top of my foot. A moment later, I sat at my desk, chair tilted back and feet up, and smiled, having finally, escaped.

BOBBY

The count, instead of lasting the usual 15 or 20 minutes, slogged on interminably for over an hour. Ordinarily, that wouldn't have mattered; but knowing Bobby was to be released soon, I was anxious to resume our rap.

In our many long conversations, Bobby had made me aware of my inadequacies as a human being: not only a racist, I was a coward, unable to face professional and social stresses, who, instead of dealing directly with the actual causes of my anger and frustrations, used narcotics as an escape.

The delay was due to the absence of two of our people, and no one could move until they either showed up on their own or were tracked down. Ultimately, the AWOLs were discovered wandering aimlessly near the gazebo: sweating, shaking, and slobbering. One said he thought he was dying, the other, going crazy, and both were screaming about *hearing* bright colors and *seeing* ear-piercing sounds. It was obvious they had dropped acid, and were having a trip that soon went from bad to worse by their being dragged off and thrown into the blackness of isolation. The rumble was they had licked "electric Kool-Aid" off the back of a postage stamp.

When I finally caught up with Bobby in the cafeteria, he was reading a letter from the U.S. Parole Commission. When I scanned his good news, I became flushed with confused emotions. I was happy for him, but envious. It hurts to watch someone, especially a friend, being set free, when you're still caged like an animal.

I asked him to tell me more about his life. I needed to know his story.

With his eyes half closed and his feet perched on the table top, he continued: "After my folks were lynched, I was damned to living in and escaping from nigger orphanages bossed by sadistic crackers. We slept on broken down cots in dorms housing 40 or 50 kids, half of whom were always sick with somethin' or other. We ate slop, and if you didn't eat every bit that was set in front of you, you didn't eat the next day. We boogied our asses off scrubbin' floors, cleanin' toilets, doin' laundry, and whatever. We sweated in the summer and froze in the winter. I don't know why, but, those Georgia nights could sure get cold . . .

"The worst of it, though, was those fuckin' booty bandits who liked to use little colored boys. My butt still aches when I think of 'em. Some of 'em tore my butt up so bad, my shit was full of blood for weeks, and the pain, so bad, I purposely wouldn't eat for days, so I wouldn't have to take a dump.

"I slipped away from the last one, somewhere up near Athens, when I was 16, still under the impression my name was 'Boy.' I got a hold of some cash by stealing the wallet of one of the chicken hawks after he had had his way with me in his office. It had dropped on the floor while he was pulling up his pants. There was 30 bucks in it which was enough to get me goin' for a while. I hitched my way to LA 'cause I heard niggers were getting a fair shake out there. I got a job for a while as a Stepin Fetchit extra for Universal Studios, mostly doing jungle films.

"The bottom line was, I ended up doin' nigger work, loadin' and unloadin' trucks for UPS, while going to night school. After I got my GED, I moved up to Oakland and went to Merritt College. It's a small hick college that takes students without a high school diploma. There were a lotta blacks in 'Oaktown,' and a pretty decent number in the college which, I guess, is why they offered a few courses in Afro-American studies, and if you were a California resident, there was no tuition.

"But I never got a degree. In my freshman soch course I met two brothas, Huey Newton and Bobby Seale, and we started to hang together. Turns out they were the big cats in the Merritt 'Triple-A,' the Afro-American Association and asked me to join. There were about 25 of us, maybe five or six girls, all from the bottom of the economic pyramid. We'd meet maybe once or twice a week at the Mau Mau, a local juke joint, where we'd sit around drinking Colt 45s, and rappin', mostly 'bout how all the white kids were making it, and we were still running around in circles. After a few 45s, we were ready to take on the world.

"At the meetings, we'd listen to tapes or watch movies of our idols: guys like Malcolm X, H. 'Rap' Brown, Erika Huggins, and Nikki Giovanni hammering away to get the vanillas off their collective inertia when it came to civil rights, and that we needed to be on the offensive. They all believed that a militant showdown was the best solution. We agreed. We were fed up with waiting. We were tired of being pushed around, tired of being poor, tired of being out of work, tired of living in ghettoes, tired of waiting . . .

"Let's see . . . where was I? Oh, yeah, I think it was around September in 1966 when one of our rat pack heard of some group in Alabama whose name I can't remember. Anyhow, they felt that working with whites was dangerous, and any commitment to nonviolent action, suicidal. Their idea was to use militant tactics to achieve political power. To us, their idea of arming themselves was an inspiration. It fired us up, as did their symbol, a snarling, black panther. We thought it could be our way of carrying out Malcolm's work. A month later, in the Student Union over at Merritt, we snuck in a case of Colt 45 and a truck-load of pizzas, and kicked off the Black Panthers. We really believed it would shake off our white albatross.

"We weren't interested in Martin's integration bullshit. We didn't want to be whitened. We were not going to *politely* request equality. We were going to *demand* it. It was going to be like Eldridge said, 'Total victory for black people or total destruction for America.' It was as simple as that."

HANNAH

Dr. Fromm had Hannah seen by a neurologist, who, after a thorough physical examination, a spinal tap, and a CT scan, concurred with the diagnosis of a major depressive episode.

One Saturday morning after two weeks of unsuccessful treatment, Dr. Fromm told me she had just finished presenting Hannah's case at the Saturday morning psych conference, and everyone felt that the only thing left to do was electroconvulsive therapy.

Shaken and scared, all I could say was, "Oh, my God, oh, my God, shock therapy?"

Hannah's brain resisted the electricity at first, but after the eighth time Dr. Fromm positioned the flat, disc-like electrodes on her shaved temples, and for a second or so zapped her with 150 joules of live, hot current, something happened. The instant the current surged through her brain, every single muscle in her body convulsed, all at once. She became stiff, her body assuming the shape of a crescent. In a few seconds, the rigidity subsided, and for 20 or so seconds, every muscle in her body began to jerk uncontrollably, and then, nothing. She was in a coma. It was as if her brain had gone up in smoke.

Hannah was never the same. The essence of her inner self had been burned out. She lost her enthusiasm for life. She just went through the motions automatically and woodenly, like a robot.

Not only had the chemistry of her brain been altered, but the chemistry between us was as well. She was indifferent, to the point of being glacial toward me. What passion she had left was reserved entirely for our boys. Her relationship with them was the antithesis of that with me. She remained, just as before, a sensitive, serious and devoted mother, becoming an intimate and intrinsic part of every facet of their lives. I, as well, wanted to be something of consequence in their lives, if only to vicariously capture what had eluded me when I was a child. But Hannah shielded them from me, and, ultimately, when she insisted on my moving out, my children and I became distant as well.

Cast aside as a husband and as a father, I was no longer a leading man, but rather a supporting character in all their lives. Before long, this unappreciative little clique's use for me was only to subsidize their lifestyle. The imperious role so vital to my narcissistic personality—that I made a show of in the office and at the hospital—was repulsed at home. I wanted to escape from this meaningless marriage, but I felt trapped by the guilt of knowing I alone had made Hannah what she had become. So, unable to divorce or even separate, I withdrew into my work, where I knew I could receive from my patients the mass adoration I so needed. I may have lost the love of my wife and children, but I knew I still had my dual love affair with Maggie and Demerol.

BOBBY

When Bobby had finished eating, he was called in to see the warden. The whisper was he was being sprung that day. After more than 4,000 days of waiting, he was, at long last, goin' home. This once-proud Panther was being set free.

I walked with him, in silence, as far as the guard tower. He set down his bag, and we just looked at each other, neither of us quite knowing what to say. Before either of us could think of anything, Orville Taggart began screeching from the window of the prison Plymouth curbed on the other side of the tower gate, "Leth get a move-on! You're gonna mith the buth!" Shaking our heads and laughing, Bobby and I impulsively hugged each other, and shook hands. "Take it to the limit, brotha," he said to me, flinging his bag over a shoulder. He didn't look back.

As the prison van faded around the bend, a distinct sense of loss suddenly possessed me. It was a strange feeling, saying good-bye like this to someone who had enriched my life in so many ways. Perhaps, my first friend.

For about an hour, I stood staring at the road, feeling more alone than I could ever remember. I probably would have lingered in that spot all day had not the guard in the tower fixed the laser beam of his rifle on my heart and yelled down, "Hey, asshole! Disappear!" I slowly shuffled back to my bunk, barely aware of who or where I was.

CHAOS

The Demerol, now in complete control of my life, was taking less and less time to wear off. My bodily responses to this raging need provoked wild mood swings—from euphoria to rage—that not infrequently caused patients to complain or suddenly vanish from inside an examining room. It was usually the complex patients with complex problems who did so, inasmuch as I no longer had the time, patience, or mental capacities to deal with them. I was pleased when they left and went elsewhere, especially when I was coming down.

My medical practice turned to chaos: an appointment schedule that had become a mishmash; careless piles of messy, undictated charts scattered everywhere; patients in gowns peeking out of doorways, wondering when I was coming back to finish their exam, not realizing I had completely forgotten they were there, or that I was locked in my office, asleep, with a syringe stuck in my thigh, or had gone to the "storeroom" with Maggie.

Before Maggie entered the picture, I was kept busy enough at the Good Samaritan Hospital, and was making enough money in my office that I resigned from the staffs of the other three hospitals where I had privileges. It was getting to be too much, especially the driving, not to mention the interminable intrusions during our nocturnal, "jag" parties. But, as fate—or rather Demerol—would have it, even one hospital proved too much, and the situation there deteriorated in sync with the office.

Whereas doctors traditionally make their hospital rounds early in the morning, primarily to get that bother out of the way, I usually coasted in around midnight, looking like hell but all hopped up and rarin' to go. The graveyard, nursing shift—most of whom were asleep on their feet—after being stunned out of their lethargy by my sudden intrusion would stare with heavy eyes, silently and unbelievingly, as I noisily pulled the metal-jacketed charts out of the rack—not infrequently the wrong ones—clattered complacently down the corridors that had been dimmed and silenced for the night; woke up patients—not infrequently the wrong ones—who, finally, after their usual, aggravating, hospital day had gratefully swallowed their "sleepers" and were now snoring; wrote orders—not infrequently inappropriate, illegible, or in the wrong chart; or even discharged patients, right then and there.

When I got back to the office after making rounds, I would, on occasion, completely forget I had been at the hospital, and go back. When I reentered the floor I would often hear a disparaging, "Oh, shit, he's here again." After which, the charge nurse, with a forced smile, would ask, mockingly, "Did you forget to do something, Doctor?"

Once, after pinning an 80-year-old's fractured hip, I left her to her own means for six days before the super gently reminded me of her presence, and that, perhaps, it was time to send her back to the nursing home. Thank God I had remembered to perform the surgery! During those days, I was forgetting a lot of things, but the one thing I never forgot was Demerol.

Again, no one seemed interested in or concerned about the reason for my inappropriate behavior, not even in the OR where it could only be described as potentially deadly. Every time a scrub tech put a scalpel in my hand, I was making book on myself.

The minor cases posed no problem. But, the major cases—spines and hips, often lasting several hours—were another story. They would start out great, since after my wakeup jab I would be in a state of euphoria—calm, steady, and a pleasure to work with. After a couple of hours, however, when the level of drug was on the wane, I would become agitated and testy, especially if things weren't going well. I would snap at the nurses, throw instruments and tantrums that would often send a nurse or tech out of the room fuming or in tears. But, that behavior, again, was not really taken seriously. Hell, lots of surgeons behaved that way. It was almost considered routine.

But it wasn't routine for a surgeon in the midst of a major operation to get nauseous, or to start breathing heavily, or to fumble due to shaking hands, or to sweat on the patient, or to take a break and just leave the room in order to take a hit. The craving and the withdrawal would become too much, and I couldn't go on without refueling. Acting as if I had suddenly come down with cramps and needed to rush to the bathroom, I would break scrub. Under cover of a stall, I would shoot up from a loaded syringe I had concealed under my shirt, flush, and get back to the case—a changed man—ready, once again, to save lives.

Before long, everyone in that OR, in fact, everyone in that whole hospital, and probably everyone in the county knew something was wrong with me, and that that something was drugs. Yet, no one made any effort to take the scalpel out of my hands until I had crippled too many bodies and lives.

Less than one year after entering the solo practice of orthopedic surgery, I received a certified letter from the chief of staff politely informing me that I was being suspended from the medical staff of the Good Samaritan Hospital because of all things, my failure to complete medical records and my lack of attendance at required meetings. It was not because I had become a menace. I was certain the hospital was harboring the hope that this disciplinary action would, somehow, cause me to vanish from their elite ecosystem, in which case, they would not have to deal with the brutal truth. They took the safe way out.

TIME

In this rigid and structured domain called prison, time slowed down, agonizingly. Time, which I had always visualized as being a fast-moving straight line with starting and ending points, became a languishing zigzag.

Outside there was never enough time, everyone was always at war with time, always in a rush, always afraid of being late, always looking at their watches, always angered at everyone else's inertia. Time flees out there like a vein shot of Demerol. I grieved a lot at first while working on my hands and knees about having to waste this relativity called time before waking up to the fact I had been given a precious gift in which to search for peace. It began to dawn on me that this was golden time, not to be wasted. God knows, I'd wasted enough.

With that end in view, I set about seeking opportunities to feast on time, to do things that might provide intellectual, psychical, and spiritual bread for my soul. I would allow time to heal, rather than destroy.

It was a gift only God could give.

My gift was empowering me to saw through the emotional bars that had always held me captive. They were solid, case-hardened, intransigent bars, but I had the time to keep sawing and sawing—while eating, while buffing, while running, while cleaning, while soul-searching, while remembering.

LAST CHANCE

At times, I tried to cut down, but I just couldn't stop completely. The will power, the moral fiber, the courage, just wasn't there. Demerol had completely destroyed any common sense I may once have had that would have allowed me, at least, to ask for help. Since I couldn't stop completely, I knew I couldn't stop working. I was hurting for money. Without money, there would be no drug, and I couldn't let that happen.

When I realized money was becoming pretty damn scarce, pretty damn quick, I began to panic. I needed to get some patients, and I needed a hospital to put them in. And, I needed to do it soon. I already owed Vern and Elaine back pay, and Hannah owed Lourdes. But the biggest fear for me was not being able to get my panacea without pesos.

There was one hospital in the immediate area I was confident would take me on: Lincoln Memorial in Alexandria. It was a small, three-story, non-descript, austere-looking, brick building, with only 40 beds. It was wholly owned by a wealthy Romanian immigrant surgeon who, before converting what had been a condemned, apartment building into a hospital of sorts, had been, like me, booted out of every hospital in the area. In his case, it was for operating on anyone for anything—from abortions to brain tumors—whether they needed it or not.

Somehow at our first brief meeting this old-world charmer never got around to asking why I wanted to be a member of his staff. He just mentioned there weren't any orthopods on his staff and asked me when I could start.

This was it: my last chance. If I screwed up here, I would no longer be allowed to practice medicine. Not that I really wanted to. I'd thought of leaving the profession, but what could I do for a living? I couldn't afford to retire; an infinite quantity of drugs, an apartment, an office, and a family costs money. Hannah had not asked for a divorce or even a legal separation. She didn't seem to care. Her children were her life, and she knew I would never forsake her or them, at least financially.

NEW FRIENDS

The prison library was a small boxy room with walls of unrelieved somber-gray cinder blocks, and although austere—a couple of tottering tables with mismatched chairs, six or seven school desks (the kind with an attached arm) and a blackboard, and all covered with graffiti—it was friendly.

Unfortunately, there was no cozy nook in which to curl up with a good quiet read and a hot cup of tea. Often, the musty odor, the chipped plaster, and the billowing spider webs would transport me back to that seedy *heder* in Cleveland, Ohio.

The few shelves that held an eclectic jumble of battered, yellowing, food-stained books (which I was given permission to inventory and systematize) were encased in glass cabinets. On Saturday mornings from eight to nine, the administrator would unlock these cabinets and allow his house guests to check out no more than two books which had to be returned the following week.

There was a fair selection of Gunthers, Louie L'Amours, and Micheners, a few legal texts, several Bibles and Qurans, and a few Stephen Kings. And although there was a shelf bursting with books pertaining to the African-American experience, I seldom saw a black inmate check them or any other book out.

There were also several masterpiece novels—Jane Austen's Pride and Prejudice, Charlotte Brontë's Jane Eyre, Ann Tyler's The Accidental Tourist, George Eliot's Silas Marner, and John Fowles' The Magus—that dealt with lost, despairing souls who succeeded in overcoming their psychic conflicts by undergoing a process of transformation through confrontational and tender interactions. They were powerful, literary perceptions—therapeutic narratives—of what healing is.

It was heartening to read about successful change and new beginnings particularly when encountering shocking revelations that hit home like Elizabeth Bennet's in <u>Pride and Prejudice</u>, "Till this moment, I never knew myself."

These, my new found friends, by transporting me to better worlds, helped keep me sane. They gave me freedom and peace.

Reading, like any blissful, enlightening adventure, soon became addictive. Kafka's portraits of tormented souls struggling to come to terms with an absolute power while imprisoned by guilt and anxiety in a hostile world became my passion, and a surprising find, Freedman and Kaplan's psychiatric text, my surrogate Bible.

The latter had the effect of routinely turning my literary chapel into a clinic in which I was both the psychiatrist and the patient. Before long, the two of us, as a result of my eagerness to enter into a metamorphosis, blossomed into a robust, synergistic, and honest relationship. We both knew, however, it would not be an easy task to free myself from myself. It would take time and perseverance to excavate the untold number of emotional bricks, crusted with pain and disappointment that had paved my road to damnation.

THE DEA

That there was such a thing as a Drug Enforcement Administration task force in the state of Virginia never once entered Maggie's or my mind. But I soon learned there was one, in Richmond, a good one, whose aggressive agents, in the never-ending fight against drugs, went from one end of the state to the other tracking down doctors who over-prescribed or abused "controlled dangerous substances:" narcotics, tranquilizers, and amphetamines.

One morning, as Elaine was unlocking the door to the office, she noticed a well-dressed, young "cowboy" leaning against the nearby wall smoking a briar pipe. After their eyes met, he reached in his jacket pocket and flipped open a leather wallet to expose a bright, gold shield.

While the narc waited, Elaine ran to the back to look for me. Not finding me in my office, she furiously pounded on the bathroom door, right in the midst of my wake-up injection. "Hurry up," Elaine whispered, "there's some guy with a big, gold badge in the waiting room."

After asking who I was and showing me his badge, the agent asked to see my controlled substance log and the charts of all the patients listed in it.

I told him I never kept a log and I didn't know I had to. And then, with a sudden burst of Demerol bravado, I asked, "Do you have a subpoena for such documents?"

"No, sir. At this time I don't. I was hoping to keep this informal."

The following week a sheriff showed up. He blandly read me my rights, and informed me he would forego the cuffs if I gave my word I would appear at the D.A.'s office for questioning.

With the help of a clever lawyer whom I had done some personal injury for, the D.A. agreed to drop the case. But the DEA agent refused to budge from his demand that the State Board of Medicine be notified.

Nine months later, when the medical board finally got around to my case, I learned that its members, instead of protecting the public from physicians like me, let me off easy.

I also learned that there is not only one, but two medical boards: one, composed of all the board members, that holds open, public meetings and hearings; the other, a hush-hush, judiciary panel made up of two or three board members that negotiates private deals and plea bargains behind closed doors. They are able to do this because like most state, regulatory boards, they are strictly autonomous— responsible to no one. It was my cutthroat lawyer who arranged, through his "connections," to have my case heard before the "underground" board in Richmond.

The administrator of the board conducted the meeting in his private office, along with another board member, my lawyer, and a secretary who just sat there, never once lifting her pen. The whole thing took less than ten minutes. The administrator opened the meeting by telling me, "We are not trying to find any evidence to incriminate you, Doctor, since we already know, and were quite pleased to hear from the Fairfax County District Attorney that all charges against you had been dropped." He then asked, matter-of-factly, "Are you taking any of the narcotics being prescribed for office use?"

"No, sir."

With that out of the way, he told me that, by law, physicians must keep accurate logs and records of any narcotics administered to patients in the office, and that he was sure I would in the future.

"Of course, sir."

On the drive back, I kept thinking that doctors were, indeed, above the law, an opinion shared by my lawyer. During a stop for lunch, he suddenly lowered his voice and declared, "You're an addict, aren't you?"

"Why do you say that?" I asked calmly.

"When's the last time you looked in a mirror? Why don't you get some help before it's too late? Let me tell you something: if you weren't a doctor, you'd be in a jail cell right now."

It was astonishing, knowing what I was and what I had done, to have walked out of that board meeting, still free to practice my craft. Knowing, however, that I was still held in bondage—enslaved to a drug—took away any complacency or satisfaction in what had transpired.

By now, everyone—doctors, nurses, patients, the DEA, the D.A., the State Board of Medicine, the sheriff's office, my family, my employees, even the pharmacist upstairs knew something alarming was wrong with me, and that that something was most likely due to drugs. Nevertheless, no one intervened. Their apathy, it seemed to me, was as appalling as my addiction.

RELIGION

You'd think that religion, the opiate of the people, according to Marx, would especially appeal to people in prison. You'd think most prisoners—having hit rock-bottom, defeated, and suffocating in despair—would welcome religion for its soothing comfort, promises of forgiveness, offerings of a new life. But I saw who did, and those who did suffered excruciating ridicule.

The word Christian to most of the prison population was a label for a sanctimonious two-faced fraud who used religion solely for its "what's-in-it-for-me" prospects. Even the guards were of that opinion, often snickering when a Jesus freak walked by. But who could blame them? After years of contending with scores of defiant, depraved, and incorrigible jailbirds, anyone would be at a loss to believe they could be "born again."

For the most part, the skeptics were right. Those who thought the Bible route would literally set them free by swaying the parole board never imagined that its equally, self-righteous members (who saw over 80 percent of the Bible mongers they paroled at least once again) were mumbling, "Why didn't those phony Psalms singers ever go to church before? Maybe if they had, they wouldn't have ended up in this living hell."

It was a damn shame. I'm sure faith, even if it was only a psychological survival tactic, would have given many scarred souls at least a modicum of hope and the support they needed to salvage their lives. And for many, it would have acted as a surrogate for the personal attachments they had had to give up.

Chester, who had been in prison for some 21 years, told me that after finding God, he found total peace. It was hard for me to believe, but he swore that, while on the inside, he never felt as if he was missing or lacking anything in life. He believed prison was where God wanted him to be. For him, anyhow, religion was not a transparent, ephemeral scheme, it was a sublime escape.

The handful of disciples of Islam, the Muslims, often seen in their caftans and crocheted, antique-white kufis studying their green-jacketed Qurans were, however, shown consideration, if not reverence.

I once asked my friend Bobby, "Why, them?"

"Well," he told me, "you would be too if you were devoutly committed to nonviolence and were encouraged to respect people—all people—and authority. It's a great religion because it gives a person a legitimate identity, dignity, and morality. It helps the brothers in here rise above their present situation and not give up on life. It also teaches us to turn away from anything that might deter us from communing with and glorifying Allah . . . like, for instance, drugs. Oh, by the way, I hear your friend, Antoine, is converting to Islam."

MYOMODULIN

Within a span of two and a half years, I was faced with six malpractice suits. So it came as no surprise that once these legal proceedings were resolved, my insurer would have nothing more to do with me, and without insurance I would lose my hospital privileges. Having cost them a fortune, they cancelled my policy. I certainly couldn't argue with that, but, now, I had a problem: no one would insure me. So I managed to come up with a scheme to survive my malpractice crisis. It was shady, and it was fraudulent, but, being what I was, I didn't care as long as it worked.

I visited my insurance agent's office, slipped some of his blank letterhead into my briefcase when his secretary's back was turned, and used his stationery to type a letter verifying that my policy with St. Paul had been renewed. I then submitted the letter to the hospital administrator with a copy of the old policy whose dates I had indiscernibly whited out and typed over with the needed ones.

My deceit worked so well that I had the hubris to repeat this deceit for as long as I remained in practice. After all, what chance was there that someone as brilliant as I, a superb, competent surgeon, would ever get sued again?

A solution to my financial woes soon presented itself too. A pharmaceutical rep, unaware of my reputation, called to ask if I was interested in doing a Phase III study on one of his company's drugs, Myomodulin.

"Phase III," he explained, "is a clinical investigation of a drug using human subjects—the last step before submitting a drug to the

FDA for approval." He told me I'd be paid $250 per patient, plus an additional $100 for x-rays and lab work.

Two days later, the rep and the director of the company's research department arrived at my office hugging two large cartons containing the investigational drug, case report forms, informed-consent documents, and a sealed list of the contents of each container of medication, to be opened only in the event of an adverse reaction.

I had been using Myomodulin, a well-established medication, ever since my residency, and was curious to know why it was being reassessed. The director of research explained that it was a combination drug, containing a muscle relaxant, a pain killer, and caffeine. The FDA was of the opinion that the mix didn't offer patients any therapeutic advantage over taking the muscle relaxant by itself. "They presume," he divulged, "that the pain med and the caffeine don't enhance the effect of the muscle relaxant. They also feel that taking several drugs at one time increases the incidence of adverse reactions, and they're griping that patients shouldn't have to put out money for several drugs when one is enough. In fact, they've already warned us they're going to rate the drug as being only 'possibly effective' in its present form. If they do that, we're going to have to take it off the market and that would be financially disastrous. So James," he winked, "we're just going to have to show them otherwise. Aren't we?"

Each of its components, as well as the drug itself, needed to be tested along with a placebo. There would, therefore, be five sets of patients in the study. The director told me I would need 100 patients, 20 in each group, and asked if I had enough patients in my practice to complete the study within four months.

I quickly calculated the total—$30,000—and answered, "No problem."

"By the way," he added, "have you ever done any clinical research before?"

When my honest negative answer drew no response, I sensed he could care less who gave out his medication, or who was taking it. All he appeared to care about were results, and he informed me, should mine be favorable, the company would, of course, want me to continue working with them, not only on Myomodulin, but also on the development of several of the drugs in their "vast pipeline." Such work would also involve publishing papers (that they would write for me), lecturing here and abroad (at their expense of course), and participating in advertising campaigns.

No question about it, I was going to make sure that company got whatever it needed.

THE MONKEY CAGE

D oc Cav, having chanced upon me cozy in bed one rainy afternoon buried in an ancient <u>Time</u> someone had left in the toilet, assigned me to clean the visiting room, known as the "monkey cage" during the afternoons. "We don't do time in bed, here," he scolded.

Unlike the toilets, the monkey cage never became a retreat. My having no bridges to the streets made cleaning it a wistful, lonely burden that was exacerbated by having to start the task before everyone left.

The visiting room was a windowed, glaringly lit yet dreary, somber-grey bunker in which 27 card tables and 76 folding chairs were overseen by a squad of surveillance cameras and a flock of hacks stationed behind a counter.

It was a highly emotional theatre, wet with the tears of those who were made to do time as well—wives, girlfriends, parents, children—and charged with tortured looks, poignant pouts, pathetic moans, and convulsive sobs.

It was agonizing to watch these pathetic souls trying to squeeze a week, a month . . . a year . . . of flesh and blood with all its passions into a few hours: playing cards, watching TV, joking, cuddling, crayoning, nursing babies, going over report cards, or feasting on KFC while locking hands or fondling each other under draped coats. The cons were filled with dreams and promises, expressed with all the sweetness and sincerity they could muster. *"As soon as I get out, hon, I promise we're gonna do this, we're gonna do that, we're goin' here, we're goin' there, we're gonna buy this, we're gonna buy that. I'll make it up to you. I swear to God."*

As I watched them, I wondered what I'd say to Hannah if she ever came to visit, or even if she were ever to accept my collect calls.

I never gave you anything but heartache, did I Hannah? You and everyone else. I'm so sorry. I'm sorry I caused you so much misery in the past. But, darling, we can have a future. I know now how precious life is, and I don't want to miss any more of it, and I don't want to miss it without you. Here, in this crowded emptiness, life is a melting dream of sadness and despairing loneliness, one that I know I'll never return to. As soon as I get out, hon, I promise.

MYOMODULIN

alsifying entire investigational studies is no easy matter. But I did it, and I got away with it for a long time by deceiving, defrauding, and betraying so many. It was easy to get patients to be included in the study. Sometimes I would select names from the patient files in the office, or use names listed in the telephone book, or in the obituaries of the <u>Washington Post</u>, or just make them up. The protocol, however, required each patient to sign an informed consent that outlined the facts of the study, including the likelihood of receiving a placebo instead of actual medication, and, of course, the risks involved, including death. The solution to the signature problem was easy. I forged them—over 2,000 before being collared—counterfeiting some with my right hand, others with my left.

To obtain blood tests and x-rays for my spurious patients, all I had to do was use the printed forms from the Lincoln Hospital lab or x-ray department. All of the doctors there were given blank forms on which they checked off the tests or the particular x-rays their patients needed. I went one step further. I wrote in the results.

What at first seemed to be an insurmountable problem, however, but which soon proved to be easy too, was deciphering exactly what bottle contained what in order to determine what each of my fictitious patients was receiving. That, of course, was essential in making sure those receiving the true drug had the highest percentage of effectiveness. Each bottle had been labeled with a coded number, the actual identity of which had been listed and sealed in an envelope. It was an envelope that wasn't an envelope, for it hardly kept its contents secret. I discovered that fact after rummaging through the study supplies and chancing upon the sealed envelope. It was a joke: a thin, brown envelope containing a single sheet of unfolded paper upon which the key had been typed, and, which, by holding up to the light, became so legible I didn't even have to squint to read it.

Now that I knew what each of my "patients" was taking, I could fabricate the case report forms for each group in a statistically meaningful way, making sure that at least a majority of the patients, perhaps 50 to 60 percent, had some effect from the individual active components of the drug when taken separately, whereas, only 20 to 25 percent of the placebo group found happiness with what they were taking. On the other hand, at least 85 percent of those taking the combination drug were written up as having had excellent relief of their symptoms.

Less than four months after my entry into the field of clinical research, I was celebrating the completion of my "important contribution to the field of medicine," and arranging for the next series of patients—this time 200. With a check for $33,000 in my pocket for perhaps 25 hours of creative albeit criminal work, I was, to be sure, more than eager to resume.

CONFRONTATION

Searching out and taking on one's false-self is a turbulent affair, an intensely disturbing confrontation. Until then, the two of us had never been conversant—or even acquainted—so, as expected, our confrontation proved to be dramatic.

At first my attempts yielded nothing but shadows, but after what seemed like interminable soul searching, revelatory flashes of the screwed-up childhood that had forged my false-self, which ultimately led me to hit rock bottom, began to appear. And then one day, they broke through.

I was outdoors, jogging around the muddy track during a violent thunderstorm, when I confronted my demons in full force. All of my ugly, unresolved conflicts—my insecurity, inferiority, unlovability— rose up and struck me like lightening bolts. Suddenly I saw myself for what I was: a soul overburdened with contemptible, shameful sin.

This truth set me free. I realized I was now free to scrutinize, upgrade, and improve my life. I could learn to respect and value my life and thus live at peace with myself. I began to see change. I could look at myself in the mirror without flinching. Most importantly, I began to repossess my own mind. Clearheadedly, I began to search for answers to long overdue questions, such as "Who am I?" and "Where do I belong?"

MYOMODULIN

It took less than six months to finish the 200-patient Myomodulin study. Upon receipt of the last case report, the director of research handed them over to the company's analysts who, after their assessments of the contained data were, to say the least, ecstatic. The finalized tabulations were then hand carried to the FDA headquarters in Rockville, Maryland.

Three weeks later, "owing to the highly creditable data submitted," the FDA changed the rating of Myomodulin from possibly effective to substantially effective.

The news of this coup spread through the industry like wildfire. Everyone, including the CEOs of the company, I was told, was pleased with my work, a paper would be published, and I would soon be receiving materials for a Phase III study on a potential anti-inflammatory drug tentatively labeled, Myosen. They assured me they were looking forward to my continued testing of their drugs on as many patients as possible, "just to make our friends at the FDA happy." If only they knew that I had, at the tips of my fingers, an infinite number of human volunteers, and could, therefore, participate in any number of clinical investigations all at the same time.

Shortly after this company's upset victory, I was literally besieged with calls from other pharmaceutical firms imploring me to perform clinical trials on their pipeline drugs. It was unbelievable: monumental firms with monumental rivalries, and monumental money. This money proved way too attractive to spurn, especially since the newer drugs, having only a single, active constituent, were easily tested.

Only two sets of patients were required: one taking the active drug, the other, of course, the placebo.

At times, I was doing three or four different studies at the same time. No doctor on this planet ever had that many patients, but not a single firm, while knowing full well of my eclectic research, ever bothered to question or attempt to find out exactly what was going on. I was giving them exactly what they needed to help ensure FDA approval, future profits, and gratified shareholders.

And they were giving me what I needed. I was making a fortune, sending most of it to an off-shore, tax-free haven. At the rate things were going, I would have enough money within two or three years to lock in a life spent rocking in a hammock set between two palm trees on the platinum sands by the sapphire waters of the Caribbean.

TOILET R&R

Several times a week, after lights out, a clique of badass blacks, ignoring the stench and the presumptuous vermin, commandeered the toilet and transformed it into a hangout for a diversity of clandestine "escapes."

It was a psychological niche—a hiding place—where they could live as individuals on their own terms: a slice of home that provided a haven from the stress and conflict of mainline prison with its razor fences and its "eyes" standing in dog houses high above you no matter where you turn. "I repeat, gentlemen, we do NOT give you the privilege of a warning shot."

Just in case the screws on duty during "business hours" weren't playing the game or weren't being "greased," a lookout was needed. Traditionally, the "Lord of the Loo," regardless of color, got to be the "hawk." The job was a godsend, for its honorarium, apart from scraps of "liberated" food and the privilege of killing time with BMOCs, proved priceless: protection. Never again did anyone press me for coins or toiletries, or miraculously crack open my locker without trashing the padlock. And I slept a lot better on the assumption the protection included Antoine.

Other than the times the babyfaced new fish were being gang-banged into ass peddlers, being the silent eye for the hangout turned out to be enlightening to me.

It was usually around eight that the brothers trooped in, made themselves comfortable on the thrones or on a few borrowed chairs, set up a card table or two, and forgot time. Against a background of doo-wop, they amused themselves rapping, playing cards, flipping slowly through tattered smut mags, burning tea, getting inked (tattooed) with a Paper Mate pen wired to a battery, or drinking pruno, a homemade wicked kick in the guts that tasted like a martini made out of piss. Such evenings soon became indispensable monotony breakers.

At other times, the toilet was turned into a chow wagon where the cheese sandwiches, toasted with a clothes iron, and the scrambled eggs, fried in a dustpan, were a delight, but the *tour de force* were the snatched slabs of steaks known as stakinies. Held in bent clothes hangers, they were roasted like marshmallows over a make-do camp stove fashioned out of a dustpan fueled with loosely rolled-up toilet paper donuts. The blackening, sputtering meat quickly suppressed the prevailing odor with a sublime fragrance, and the crusty, dripping chunk thrown my way, proved divine.

Engrossed in their doings, no one took notice of the dopers who came in to shoot up using broken eye droppers, or to sniff varnish stolen from the furniture shop. Whatever poison they polluted their bodies with, however, worked. After a while everyone seemed to be nodding or purring like kittens. "Hey, Doc, try some. It's a swell way to end the day."

"Yeah, don't I know, but thanks anyhow."

The protection "cush," thank God, proved real.

I remember it was sometime in February because I was seated on a foldaway leaning ambivalently against the door jamb reading a piece in a week-old Richmond Times-Dispatch about Jean Harris being convicted of murdering the Scarsdale Diet doctor. Feeling a shadow, I looked up. Rather than the expected, questioning guard, there was a lewdly grinning, black human mountain reeking of body odor and Old Spice caressing a needle-pointed screwdriver.

"C'mon inside, punk," he whispered hoarsely, "I wanna shove my dick up your ass."

"Oh, really?" I snickered in mortal fear as I tried to remedy my teetering chair.

"Yeah, really," he said, just as Kareem grabbed his wrist.

IMPENDING DOOM

With few exceptions, the better-known pharmaceutical firms who asked me to work for them were honest and aboveboard, all having a national network of sincere, clinical investigators who were testing the same drugs as I. Because of that, I was careful not to submit results that might arouse suspicions of impropriety. For the sake of credibility, I always made sure some of the patients never returned, had allergic reactions, slightly abnormal lab results, or innocuous complications like nausea and vomiting. And I always threw in a few with such psychosomatic symptoms as impotence, choking, or chest pain, all of which were believable, and to be expected in those taking any drug or a placebo.

A few of the firms kept the list of what each patient was taking at their headquarters with instructions to call an emergency number should the need arise. Most, however, had the key to the bottle codes sealed in some sort of tamper-proof wrapper. Despite that, determining what was in each bottle proved to be a simple matter, since placebos dissolved in hot water, whereas the drugs didn't. They required some sort of organic solvent like alcohol. Occasionally, all I needed to do was taste: the placebo was sweet; the drug, bitter.

The drug firms couldn't have been more delighted with the results of my deception. In compliance with FDA regulations, they would send monitors over periodically to review my work and pick up completed forms. All of these monitors were interested in only one thing—numbers. They all wanted to accumulate, in the shortest period of time, as many patients as possible who had shown a positive response. All of them were knocking themselves out to be the first to get their anti-inflammatory, analgesic, or muscle relaxant approved before the competition. No one seemed even remotely concerned over the possible existence of duplicitous clinical trials.

But I was doing too much wrong, too fast. Within three years, I had participated in at least 20 clinical investigations involving upwards of 2,000 patients, all the while throwing caution to the wind, for I knew damn well the FDA was aware of my involvement since every New Drug Application (NDA) submitted to them was accompanied by a list of the clinical investigators that had been contracted to perform the Phase III trials. My truly audacious display of bravura and deceit may very well have been caused by greed and sophistry, and the result of a mind maimed by drugs and insanity. It could also have been a hidden desire to be caught. That way I would be freed of the angst and loneliness that were making me loathe myself and wish I were dead.

Sometime in September of 1977 my name happened to cross the desks of the FDA once too often. Finally raising suspicions, it touched off a blitzkrieg of an investigation that made my life even more wretched than it already was.

The first bomb fell in the boardroom of a small pharmaceutical firm based in New Jersey. The six clinical investigators, including myself, who had participated in the Phase III studies of their hoped-for anti-inflammatory drug, Astrocin, had been invited to review the statistical analyses of our case studies prior to the submission of the NDA to the FDA. The drug had been proven to be exceptionally effective with only a minimum of side effects, all minor. Everyone was excited, not only because of the results, but because, if the drug was approved, it would be the first non-steroidal anti-inflammatory on the market, and would make this small company a real player in the pharmaceutical world.

It was during a coffee break that the vice-president of the company searched me out. He found me in a corner, alone, drinking coffee. After congratulating me on my work, he mentioned that he had recently spoken to the Commissioner of the FDA and the director of its Bureau of New Drugs, both of whom indicated they would personally be involved in the review of the Astrocin NDA, if for no other reason than the entire project, from the lab to the public, had, inconceivably, been completed in less than two years which was, frankly, unheard of.

He also mentioned they were quite aware of my work as a clinical investigator and were particularly interested in the results of my Astrocin study, since, of the 500 patients that were treated with the drug, 240 had come from my office. The bottom line was they were sending a "crackerjack" investigative team to my office within the next couple of weeks to go over my research. He asked me if I'd ever been audited before. When I answered no, he said not to worry about it. He was sure my work would pass the closest scrutiny, as he had been quite impressed by the detailed, case study reports I had submitted, every one of which, he had personally reviewed.

As he spoke I broke out in a cold sweat and could feel my heart begin to race and my stomach ignite. I was stunned: paralyzed with panic. I felt as if I was going to pass out. I didn't want him to say any more. I couldn't bear what he was telling me, so I excused myself by telling him I thought the meeting was about to resume, and I still needed to go to the bathroom.

I ran out of the boardroom furiously looking for the men's room. After finding it and thanking God it was empty, I ran into a stall, bent over, and retched the very lining of my stomach into the toilet. I stood up trembling, seeing flashes and feeling as if a pile driver was thumping inside my skull. I needed a shot, but all I had with me were three tablets of Demerol wrapped in a piece of toilet tissue tucked in my wallet. I gulped them down with a handful of water from the sink, managing to get the entire front of my suit and tie wet.

That night the shameful wrong of what I had been doing for so long finally erupted through the muck and the mire of my Demerol-addled brain. I became frantic with the realization of my unpardonable criminality. My mind went in circles. I thought of arguing insanity and confessing: making known the truth as to precisely who and what I was. Sure then everyone in the world would know, including the police! This time they'd throw the book at me. No! I couldn't let anyone know. No one. The anxiety of such a confession would be devastating. My ego could not tolerate failure.

So I continued my voyage of deceit, fueled by Demerol and my lust for riches that had taken hold of me as strongly as the drug ever had. I had no idea I was no longer in control: no longer rational, no longer sane. I was possessed by Demerol. And so, faced with an insurmountable problem, it was the Demerol that came up with the solution.

FISHING

It was one of those sunny days that had the power, even in a penitentiary, to profoundly change one's temperament.

I was scrubbing the floor in the toilet when Cavendish sauntered in, surprise in hand, and announced that it was a day made to order for fishing.

"Hey, Doc, put down the brush! Go dig up a few worms."

When I admitted to Cav I'd never once fished and didn't know how, he stared at me incredulously, shrugged his shoulders, and then tossed me the rod. It was a bright blue affair, with a lump of lead, a red-and-white float, and a few good-size hooks.

"All you gotta do," he demonstrated, "is stick a worm on the hook like so . . . cast it in the water . . . wait 'til it moves . . . give it a little yank . . . then reel 'er in."

He was right. That was the gist and the simple joy of it, and it took me only a few casts to get the knack.

I'll never forget the rush of reeling in my first catch—a slippery catfish no bigger than my hand. And I'll always remember removing the hooked worm from that fish's gaping, gasping mouth and gently returning it to the water, where, after a moment of confusion and a quick snap of its tail, it swam deep to freedom.

Had I not caught anything, it still would have been a sublime experience, for the bliss of fishing, I soon discovered while waiting for the next tug, is not necessarily found at the end of the line. It can be found in the Zen-like peace that comes with watching the float bobbing in the eddies, squinting at the sun's twinkling reflection on the water, listening to the birds trilling in the surrounding trees.

I had come to that lazy stream that day to savor, at least, solitude. I'd needed to brood and continue my ongoing soul-searching. But I found more there. Becalmed by my newfound pastime, grief and despair were banished. In their place, I saw hope. As I waited for another fish to bite, I envisioned a future filled with simple joys, such as these. Someday—soon—I told myself, I'd be able to take my sons fishing.

After a few hours, my reverie was shattered by a familiar voice. "GET YOUR FUCKIN' ASS UP HERE, BOY!" the hack bellowed, "AND I MEAN PRONTO!"

I quickly swooped up my fishing gear and kicked myself up the steep path towards the apoplectic guard. I'd missed the damn count.

MACHIAVELLIAN MACHINATIONS

Demerol's solution seemed simple: destroy the evidence. So, five days before the invasion, I gathered all 2,000 or so case reports from all the clinical investigations I had ever done. In a state of restrained frenzy, I went through every one of them, trying to recognize the names of actual patients. I was able to identify 106. I then gathered up all the office records, both medical and financial, I could find pertaining to those names, took them back to my apartment, and pitched them in the incinerator.

Then I thought, *What if by some means—examining other office records, or hospital records, or by reviewing the consent forms given to the drug firms along with the case reports, or even going through the phone book—they somehow turned up those 106 names?* It would become readily apparent that only I would have the motive to get rid of them, and that the other 1,894 case study forms were, most likely bogus.

Before I gave them a chance to discover those discernable facts, my warped mind led me to believe I could cover up the loss of the 106 by having it appear they were destroyed along with a host of innocuous records. I had to make it look as if their total destruction was a result of a natural disaster, or by someone with a powerful motive. I certainly couldn't create a natural disaster, so that left me with the job of making it appear that the records were destroyed either by someone who desperately needed his or her records to vanish, or by someone or some organization that wanted to harm me.

Pumped full of Demerol, I rolled up my pants to mid-calf, took off my shoes, and stepped into Maggie's red stilettos she had left in the drawer with her reserve supply of panty hose. I then put on a pair of surgical gloves and hobbled to the hallway outside the office. Seeing no one, I locked the door, then forcefully jammed it open with a screwdriver. Stumbling back into the office, I systematically scattered shelf after shelf of medical and financial records, x-rays, papers, and reports all over the floor. I emptied the boxes of case study records that had been accumulating dust over the years. I then poured the contents of six, five-gallon plastic drums of x-ray chemicals over the scattered piles of medical memoirs. As the chemicals worked their corrosive magic, I stirred up the piles several times with a mop handle to make sure everything was ravaged to the point of being unsalvageable.

That done, I methodically went about with a scalpel in my hand carving swastikas on the seats and backs of all the Naugahyde-covered chairs in the waiting room, and on every one of the paintings on the walls. Then, after turning over several desks and tables, I closed the drains in all four sinks in the office and turned on the faucets of each. By that time, I was so uptight; I shot up with a huge slug of Demerol, and slumped down on the lone upright chair in the office.

After a few minutes I had calmed down enough to gather up my own shoes, the screwdriver, and the scalpel, and after putting them in an x-ray envelope with the rubber gloves I had worn during the mission, I left the building. I drove around for a while and discarded the bulging envelope, in a curb sewer, about ten miles from the office. I had done Demerol's bidding and destroyed the evidence; but I soon realized, that wasn't enough.

What I had done with the records certainly wasn't going to persuade the FDA to quash their investigation. I realized I needed to be a victim. I needed the FDA to believe I had been harmed to such an extent that I would have to retire from my medical practice. If I could convince them of that, then, maybe, not wishing to look as if they were harassing me by their investigations, they would leave me alone. And even if they did go ahead with their probe and managed to find evidence of wrongdoing, they would have mercy on me and forgo prosecution, believing I had been punished enough.

Hours before dawn on Monday morning, I took two syringes, loaded one with Novocain, the other with Demerol. After injecting the narcotic deep into the muscle of my right buttock, I numbed the skin on the top of my head with about 20 cc's of the local. When I was done contaminating my body, I discarded the syringes with their attached needles into the flame-colored, toxic waste box attached to the wall of an examining room. Slipping on a single, surgical glove on my right hand, I walked to the front door to make sure the new lock was secured, and then walked back to my office where I washed and dried my weapon of choice—an obsidian paperweight, shaped like a obelisk, which sat on my desk.

A moment later with grit and brute force, I managed to do it. As the rock-hard obsidian confronted my skull, I heard, but could not feel, the sickening crunch of bone, and the phffft of its overlying, soft tissues as they gaped open to expose the splintered, bleeding bone. As warm, viscid blood trickled down into my eyes, I could feel myself losing consciousness.

Vern found me a few hours later. He notified the ER doctor who came up with an orderly. After a perfunctory examination, they lifted me onto a gurney and wheeled me down to x-ray. A hairline fracture prompted a call the chief of surgery. While waiting, the orderly put me in a hospital gown, fortuitously leaving my under shorts on which were concealing a plethora of needle tracts; those on the rest of my body—namely my feet—went unnoticed. After the "chief," with a great deal of compassion, examined me and sewed up the jagged wound, he admitted me for observation, concerned I might possibly be bleeding within the tissues of my brain.

Other than the nausea and a brutal headache, for which they could not give me any medication on the chance it might mask the symptoms of cerebral edema or bleeding, I seemed all right. The only thing that really bothered me was the fear of withdrawal, but when Vern came down to see me just after I was admitted, he understood exactly why I needed him to go to my apartment, get the Demerol pills I had stashed, and sneak three of them to me.

Shortly after Vern left on his errand of mercy, Hannah came to visit. She had been driving her new Mercedes 450SLC over to a 7-Eleven for milk when the news of a "senseless attack on an Alexandria doctor" came over the air. She was polite but cool. She asked how I was, and if I needed anything, but didn't offer to care for me when I left the hospital. I could see she didn't want to stay, so I told her I was fine, not to worry. As she walked to the door, she turned and calmly remarked, "Oh, by the way, I don't think what you're doing is going to work, Jim. If I were you, I'd give it up."

When Vern returned with my demons, I learned how Hannah knew. After hearing of the attack, Hannah had first gone up to the office, not knowing I had been admitted to the hospital. She had arrived while the detectives were searching for clues. "When she was asking them what had happened," Vern reported, "the FDA suddenly pops in. Said they were scheduled to check on some research work you had been doing.

"Then Hannah left to come here, and the FDA guys took off on account o' the birddogs, who told 'em not to touch anything until *they* were finished with *their* work, and that it might take all day. Boy, you could tell they were pissed. They told me to tell you they'd be back. They left their card and this letter."

It was a directive from the assistant director of the Bureau of New Drugs requesting I turn over to the FDA any and all records pertaining to 800 patients I claimed had taken part in five of my clinical investigations that included the Astrocin study.

Two days later, I was released from the hospital, my head still making like a piston, but otherwise intact. The next morning, after a

Coke and some coconut cookies, I went to the office to help Vern finish cleaning up after the first incident. When I got there, I was ambushed by the detectives in the hallway outside the office. Although, it was only 8 a.m., it was apparent they had been there quite a while, as evidenced by the many scattered cigarette stubs at their feet.

After swearing I had nothing to do with either incident, they just looked at me, smoking, smirking, and shaking their heads. They made it clear they didn't believe me. "We *know*," one of them shouted, "you brought on this whole *megillah*. We know all about the FDA. This time, we're gonna get ya. That's a promise! Don't leave town!"

Three days later, as I walked out of my apartment, there they were again. This time they were more conciliatory, suggesting I take a polygraph test, "to put some closure on this case."

I knew if I refused to take the test, they would take for granted I was guilty and would then join forces with the FDA. Besides, I knew I could pass it and be rid of these Sherlocks forever. I remembered from psych that lying is an emotional provoking experience, and, as such, brings about certain physiological reactions, namely escalations in blood pressure, pulse and breathing, all of which the polygraph records simultaneously. I also knew that the physiological effects of Demerol were the exact opposite. The calming effect of the drug was the antidote to a failed polygraph, being very conducive to prevarication.

Knowing that, I shrugged my shoulders and agreed. "Of course. I'd be glad to. When?"

"Now."

"OK. Just let me go back to the apartment and call my office. I need to cancel some patients." I went back in, quickly gulped down two more "dems" to prolong the action of my wakeup shot, and ran back down.

A few days later, a follow-up piece in the newspaper about the break-ins mentioned, "the police initially suspected the doctor may have vandalized his own office . . . and had hit himself on the head, but after passing a polygraph, one of the detectives on the case said he was positive Scheiner was not responsible for the incidents." I had done it! Thanks to the Demerol, I felt invincible.

THE TOILET

I t was in the toilet where the most contemptible perversion of prison society was carried out. There, men created women out of men. The dehumanized degenerates of such wantonness were predators who used sexual violence, not only as an outlet for testosterone, but as a means of getting even for the atrocities and the injustice they had had to put up with ever since their ancestors were shanghaied out of Africa. Prison was the only place they could assert supremacy over whites. Prison was theirs. They were dubbed punks or booty bandits who lured naïve pretties into the showers, "C'mon kid, smoke a joint with us," and then proceeded to give them the surprise of their lives. To refuse the come-on meant being corralled and dragged, and then the begging, the whimpering, the scuffling, and, finally, the muffled screams. It was hard on me, and I felt the agony of it, but, like everything else, all I could do was grit my teeth and try to let it go.

And then there were the glaring drag queens. Every time you turned around, they were there with the sweet talk looking to score. "Hey, dreamboat, they tell me you're quite a stud. Wanna get it on, big boy-y?"

All it took was a buck, a "herd" of Camels . . . a Mars bar, and they dropped their pants and bent right over or got on their knees for a wham-bam-thank-you-ma'am. It was ungodly, but then, what here wasn't?

They were all uninspiring and they were all unmemorable—to me anyway—except for one, Bruce.

Kate, as he preferred to be called, spent Saturdays, his cute day, in the toilet closet after his "Daddy" helped himself to it, and with a few bed sheets, towels, a can of lavender air freshener, and a bottle of Vaseline, concocted a joy spot.

In his other life, Bruce had been a hairdresser, married, and the father of three children. Within a day of being sent up for extortion, he was gang raped. Afterwards, he came under the PC (protective custody) of a lifer known only as Ox for obvious reasons. At a prison workshop conducted by one of Ox's seasoned punks, Bruce learned exactly what he had to do in order to survive: how to use Kool-Aid for makeup, how to purse his lips, how to run his tongue around in his mouth, how to grind his ass, act shy, and even sit like a woman. When all dolled up in bikini panties, panty hose, and a padded bra, he became a stunning peroxide-blonde, chocolate drop of a trick. The lines that formed and the frequent shouts of, "Hurry up, it's my turn already," corroborated the reality of it, and implied just how well-to-do his pimp was becoming.

ERICH

An entire year passed without a word from my bureaucratic adversaries. I began to loosen up, no longer obsessed with their investigations, thinking, perhaps, the nightmare was over. I had also not heard from Vern. Why he left and where he went remained mysteries.

Conscious of the fact that the government tends to move slowly, the fact that a year had elapsed was really of no great consequence. My complaisancy, though, blew hot and cold. When cold, I gave serious thought to leaving the country. Although I had quite a bit of money concealed offshore, it was nowhere near enough to support myself and my estranged family. Even if I wanted to work as a physician out of the states, I couldn't, since medical licensing officials anywhere would require proof of my credentials, and to obtain them, I would have to contact the State Board of Medicine which meant giving my whereabouts away. I could, of course, open a bar, but that too, might attract public notice. The salaries for any other jobs I might find would probably not be worth it.

What really precluded my leaving the country was Hannah and the kids. Hannah permitted me to visit our boys, but never to be alone with them. She knew, and rightly so, I was a danger to them as long as I did drugs. Denying that I wasn't was pointless. She knew.

Most weekends, I would drop over to visit the kids bearing toys or ice cream, or both. Hannah, of course, never allowed me to drive them anywhere. A situation arose, however, when I did take Erich for a short drive.

It was on a Saturday morning when I found Lourdes, Hannah's housekeeper, alone with the twins. She explained that Hannah had flown up to Cincinnati to be with her mother who had needed emergency surgery. Erich was still at Hebrew school. Two hours later, the phone rang. It was Erich's teacher, asking me to come for Erich because the school bus broke down.

By the time I returned to the house with my son, my demon had completely taken a hold of me with frenzied claws. In my haste to rush to my office and satisfy my craving, I stopped the car, opened the back door, cautioned him to "look both ways and then run," and then allowed him to jump out and cross the street alone.

As he ran, I became conscious of a distant, reverberating rumble. Thunder? Then there was a turbulent roar, a seemingly endless screeching, a low-pitched thump, an instant of piercing silence, and a high-pitched squeal. Then the Harley roared past and blazed away into the distance, lost forever.

The crumpled, soft bundle of life landed 20 feet in front of me—face down—exactly on the white median of the black asphalt, now splattered with a spray of plum-red droplets. Paralyzed by the evil I had caused, I couldn't move until, out of the corner of my eye, I saw Lourdes, barefooted, bound out of the front door bellowing and screaming. She lovingly cradled Erich's broken, bleeding body, rocking him gently, whispering comforting words and snatches of Spanish prayers.

I don't remember the ambulance or driving to the hospital, and, only vaguely, someone in a scrub suit telling me of multiple fractures; of a hand, all but severed at the wrist; and of a face, spoiled by cruel lacerations that would take a myriad of sutures.

I do, however, remember calling to tell Hannah, and how she took the news as if she were on a first-name basis with tragedy. Before hanging up the phone, she said quietly through her tears, "Jimmy, I think it's time . . ."

I was so adamant about keeping my addiction out of the public eye that even when it became certain I was bound for prison, I kept silent. Part of me, though, wanted to go, not only for the need to suffer, but to free myself of my curse. As Hannah suggested, it was time.

Instead, within a day of the tragedy, using the standard approach of swapping one drug for another, I decided to treat myself. At about that time, propoxyphene, better known as Darvon, was becoming quite popular: at first thought to be non-addictive, but now considered a narcotic on the order of codeine. At the time, I had no idea Darvon was chemically related to methadone.

Propoxyphene is sold in various forms—pure or in combination, all of which were easily secured, since its prescriptions were never questioned by pharmacists, even if ordered 100 at a time. It wasn't at all like trying to purchase Demerol. I tried all of them, finally discovering that the seductive, gray and red capsules of Darvon Compound-65, when taken four or five at a time, made for a rather pleasant, long-lasting high: not as intense as Demerol but still, quite satisfying. During the first two weeks of the "swap," I was surprised to find the symptoms of Demerol withdrawal quite bearable, and after the third week of progressively decreasing the doses of Demerol, I was able to muddle through with Darvon, for the time being, anyhow. Of course, I was now addicted to Darvon, but, since it didn't bring about the critical diagnostic side effects of Demerol—the extreme euphoria, tremors, flushing, dizziness, sweating, and, of course the profound constricted pupils—no one could tell.

ANTOINE

As I neared the shaded track for my evening jog, I spotted a lonely figure limping near its far curve. The figure paused, listed on a cane, and turned to face me. I halted abruptly, startled, but nevertheless, pleased. It was Antoine. I had wanted to talk to him.

Since that incident in the library that had landed me in the hospital, I had been nagging myself, over and over, over what I had said about him and wishing in the worst way it had never happened. I had put myself in his place. I felt his hurt, and I hated myself for having degraded him and his race. I was disgusted over it.

An overwhelming sense of guilt and shame had swept over me, but I now knew I could shake off those twin dragons by apologizing and asking for forgiveness. Drugs were no longer an option. I smiled to myself as I resumed walking, content at being aware that it was the moral thing to do, and that I had the courage here, in this secluded wilderness, to do it. It had been bad enough telling myself, *if only I hadn't*. I didn't want to have to say anymore, *if onlys*.

I had to go through with it. If not, the angst of it would always bloody my mind. But, yet, I thought, I don't want to lose the agony of it. I need to feel it. For what I did, I damn well deserve to feel it.

When we were finally face to face, I could feel the venom of his glare. When I started to speak, "Antoine, I wanted to . . ." he grazed my stomach with the tip of his cane, curled his lips and snarled, "Go fuck yourself, peckerwood. You ain't got nothin' I wanna hear."

I wanted to hide from myself as I watched him hobble off, his cane angrily flinging divots of mud. But where? God, I felt small. I desperately wanted him to understand and to accept me as I now did him. I wanted him to accept my apology, to hear my words. *What I did was wrong. I'm sorry. Dammit, can't you see I'm sorry?*

There were so many *sorry's*—too many to count. As I continued to jog around the prison track, I thought of Hannah and the boys.

God, I wonder how they are? What do they look like? What are they doing? Oh, God, why wasn't I the one to get run over? Why him? Dammit, God! Why him?!

What do they think of me? What am I going to tell them when they ask—and they will—how I ended up here? And how am I going to ever prove to them I love them? Well . . . I'm going to tell them the disgusting truth. No more lies.

God, I wish I could be with them now: helping them with their homework, playing catch or even taking them fishing. Sometimes I wish Antoine had killed me. We'd all be better off. Maybe, if I'm lucky, he will.

THE FDA

wo weeks later, the FDA team reappeared. They swaggered in, flourishing briefcases swollen with copies of the documents they had initially asked me to produce, but because I couldn't, they had petitioned them from the drug firms.

Hunkering down, they proceeded, over the next five days, to turn my already tumultuous office upside down. For eight hours every day, except for short, brown-bag lunches and occasional coffee breaks, they looked everywhere for any records relating to any of the names I had submitted as having been included in one of the five clinical studies they were probing. They sifted through patients' charts, financial records, and appointment books: everything I hadn't destroyed. Then they went to the x-ray department and the lab.

Little by little, they found bits and pieces of evidence—charts I had overlooked, names in an old appointment book, a billing card, a lab or x-ray slip, or an insurance form with the names of actual patients I had shamelessly included in the bogus clinical investigations. All in all, enough to prove my deceit.

On Friday, just before they left, they informed me they had managed to search out 45 of the existent patients' names I had used, along with phone numbers and addresses.

And then, the calls started coming in from confused, concerned, and angry patients wanting to know who was calling them regarding some research study they were supposed to have been involved in.

These calls dragged on for two months, but the FDA team didn't come back. One month after they left, however, I received two certified letters from the directors of clinical research of two major pharmaceutical firms, for whom, even during this debacle, I was still doing Phase III trials. Both letters disclosed that their respective companies had received statements from the office of the Commissioner for Regulatory Affairs for the FDA, informing them that my privileges for conducting clinical trials of investigational drugs had been revoked, due to "professional misconduct." The directors suggested I repackage all unused drugs and other materials used in the studies and return them. The bonanza was over. A year later—just when I was beginning to think the worst was over, and that somehow the damning evidence had gotten buried in the bottom drawer of a metal desk in some stale government building—the FDA once again surfaced.

It was a Monday morning. The postman, instead of dropping off the mail, told Vern he had a registered letter that needed my signature. It was from the director of the Bureau of New Drugs informing me that according to Title 21, Code of Federal Regulations, sections 16.24 and 312.1(c) I was being notified of an opportunity for a regulatory hearing to offer an explanation, for my "deliberate and repeated violations" of the Bureau's regulations regarding clinical investigations. The letter summarized the violations as being: "failure to establish or maintain records of five clinical investigations which were, in whole or in part, never performed, as well as knowingly and willfully making false and factitious statements and representations concerning these drug studies." The hearing was scheduled for March 7, 1979.

After reading the notice, I just wanted to sleep—forever. I knew then, it was all over. Feeling obligated to brief Vern as to what was going on, I took him out for Chinese, and over a few Tsing Taos, told him everything.

After my confession, he simply said, "I'm not stupid, Doc. I knew what you'd been doin' all along."

I was sure that by now, his brain was turning into the same sort of drug-induced mush mine was, but, even so, he'd do anything for me. He loved me, and no matter what, he would always be there for me. Besides, I knew he would do anything—anything—not to lose his source. And I was his source.

After splintering open my fortune cookie, I wondered if, perhaps, there was some way Vern could help me. And then it came to me. Impetuously, I cried out, "Vern! There is something you can do. We could say we worked on these studies together. Your job being to take the data off the patients' charts and record it on the case report forms. I could say I was so busy seeing patients that I never had time to check what you had recorded. That way they'll think we actually did do the research and," I lied, "since everything was destroyed when the office was trashed, who's gonna know?"

Without a hint of hesitancy, he shrugged his shoulders and smiled, "Sure."

The hearing was held in a stale, crypt-like auditorium deep within the basement of the H.E.W. Building in Baltimore. The room could easily hold three hundred, but Vern, myself, and the compliance officer for the FDA, Frank Thomasen, were the only inhabitants that morning.

Mr. Thomasen stood on the stage behind a podium trying to transform his cherubic face into one of intimidation. After introducing himself, he explained the purpose of the hearing as an opportunity for me to explain my side of the story, to determine whether or not the case would be pursued any further, and then asked who the gentleman was seated next to me. I introduced Vern as my physician's assistant, and a participant in the clinical investigations under review. This, of course, came as a complete surprise, but Mr. Thomasen agreed to hear Vern's role in the contested research.

The young bureaucrat then wanted to know exactly how it came to be that every record pertaining to the five clinical studies under investigation were unavailable when the FDA came to my office, and whether or not they were now.

I regurgitated the details exactly as I had done to the police, but added that their investigation as well as the results of the polygraph proved I was innocent of any wrongdoing.

I had previously briefed Vern on what his supposed responsibilities as my research assistant had been, and when the compliance officer wanted to know what they were, he articulately recounted how he would have each patient sign an informed consent, how he would copy the necessary data from the patients' charts onto the case report forms, how he obtained and took the blood and urine samples down to the lab; and added, "The only thing Dr. Scheiner did was examine the patients. I did all the rest!"

Vern's statement was quite believable. In fact, so much so that Mr. Thomasen asserted he would have to amend the Notice of Hearing to include him. Whether Vern realized it or not, he had capriciously become a defendant in a rather serious, criminal affair.

During the drive home, I intuited that the hearing had been nothing but show, a legal formality. And, although Thomasen looked, spoke, and dressed like a dweeb, he was probably nobody's fool. *Dammit,* I agonized, *I should have brought a lawyer along. Even with Vern taking on part of the blame, there was no way they were going to let me get away with it with a slap on the wrist. No way! This wasn't the State Board of Medicine. These guys aren't about to take pity on us.*

Later that evening while stoned, I asked myself, *Why couldn't Vern take all the blame?*

Less than a week later, Vern received notice of his being charged with exactly the same violations that were pending against me. He was in much deeper trouble than I had anticipated, and, I was sure he hadn't the slightest idea how deep, but I was afraid if he did he would back out of his commitment, and leave me to my own fate.

I spent most of the night trying to think up ways to convince him that the allegations pending against him were of no consequence, but

I couldn't come up with anything. It didn't matter, though, seeing as how the next day, he along with the entire office stock of Pheraphen, had vanished.

BROTHER CLARENCE

Brother Clarence, the jailhouse Bible banger, had made it sound so easy. "Give your heart to Jesus," he said, "and I guarantee, just like that, you'll be purged of sin and saved."

Just like that?! Could it be that easy? Did he honestly imagine that, just like that, I could stop being a Jew, Christ would somehow enter my heart, and I'd start believing in a trinity of metaphysical absolutes? Just like that? Here? In the steel-gray and chill of a prison, a ruined life can, just like that, be made whole? Maybe for some, but dammit, I'd had enough easy solutions for one lifetime.

Clarence's devil-may-care approach to redemption, salvation, and eternal life seems wrong to me. You don't get golden honorariums, "just like that." And he's dead wrong when he said, God put me here. My God didn't make me steal zoology tests from the mimeograph room. He didn't force open my mouth and make me swallow a barge full of bennies. He didn't stick those fuckin' needles in my veins. He didn't make me wound my family. Can you imagine, my own family? My own children . . . my own wife. And, sure as hell, he didn't make me turn a simple-minded cripple into a codeine addict and then corrupt him. For God's sake, he was my friend! No! Brother, I did all that by myself.

Anyhow, how could I be converted into a Christian? My entire childhood was spent being brainwashed into believing they were the enemy and were to be hated, not only because we were better, but because they've never stopped persecuting us for praying to one God, and because *they* were brainwashed we were responsible for Jesus being crucified and doing dreadful things, like using the blood of little, Christian children in our "satanic" rituals.

But then, I thought, *why not become a Christian? I have to admit; deep down, I've always envied them. Hell, they don't have to wear freaky-looking clothes and yarmulkes. They don't have to be circumcised, and without anesthesia! And they can live wherever, go to any college, stay in any hotel, join any club . . .*

❦

Almost immediately, as Brother Clarence and his flock of three, about-to-be born-again felons, of which I was one entered the bleak but brilliantly lit Living Faith Pentecostal Church, and began tiptoeing into the furthest back pew, every head in the congregation turned sharply, and every hand impulsively reached out for the children.

There was no secret why. All you had to do was look at their faces—livid masks of repugnance and outrage—or listen to their undisguised thoughts, piqued with indignation. *How dare they come here. They're supposed to be locked up.*

It was at that moment that I knew exactly what it felt like to be a con. But just as devastating as that realization was the fact that, neither during the course of the pastor's tirade, nor during the shouting, the singing, the testimonials, and the speaking in tongues, nor after the ginger cookies and Kool-Aid had been consumed in a far-off corner did the promised revelation come to pass. There was no thunder, no exultation, no awakening, no rush, not even comfort: nothing, but guilt and anger. Clarence had lied. And so I passed on the proffered baptism which he now promised, "would surely make me see the light," and took my chances.

ATTORNEY ROTH

It had been two years since the FDA turned my office upside down looking for evidence, and I had just about convinced myself the nightmare was over. But then, on an early Monday morning, a federal marshal appeared at my office and pressed a blue-shrouded subpoena in my hand. Having done his duty, he did a snappy about-face and directed me to "have a great day, sir."

Seeing the seal of the United States imprinted on the blue jacket and below it, the words, "United States Department of Justice," I instinctively shut my eyes. The subpoena, issued by the United States District Court for the Eastern District of Virginia, was an order to appear at 10 a.m. on August 5, 1980, before a federal grand jury. I was to testify as a witness in the case of the "United States of America v. James J. Scheiner." The summons instructed me to bring any and all patient and financial records for the 800 patients listed in the enclosed computer print-out, as well as all appointment books, log sheets, ledgers, etc., for the years during which the clinical studies the FDA investigated had taken place.

I felt sick, dizzy, and weak. Crazy, blazing flecks of colors danced in front of my eyes. When the dance ended, and as I bent over the sink to rinse my mouth of the bitterness of vomit, my shoulders began jerking uncontrollably, and sweat poured down my face. After gulping a mouthful of Maalox, I locked the door, tossed down a fistful of Darvocet, and laid down on an examining table.

I knew, then, I had had enough. I couldn't go on like this any longer. I needed a lawyer, even though I knew it would be a formidable task to unburden myself to a stranger. I knew, however, I would have to, but then, pondering the prospect, I wasn't at all sure I could.

My first thought was to retain the lawyer who had defended me against the state DEA, but he was Catholic. I needed a Jewish lawyer seeing as I had intimated the vandalism to be an act of anti-Semitism, an act that only a Jew could really relate to. I hoped, too, that this fabricated act of anti-Semitism would assist my cause.

When I awoke several hours later, I opened the phone book. As I glanced through the abundance of Jewish law firms, one name stood out—Roth—Hannah's maiden name.

"Start from the beginning," Roth said, "and don't leave anything out."

⚬⚬⚬

During the recitation, I played up Vern's role, laying most of the blame on him. He took notes on his yellow legal pad then asked two questions, "What possessed you to go to Baltimore without counsel?" and "What the hell were you thinking?"

I had no answers.

"Humph," he exhaled loudly as he skeptically fixed his eyes on me, and tapped his legal pad with his pen seemingly forever before saying he would get in touch with the District Attorney's office, and for me not to worry about the grand jury, "The Fifth Amendment states you don't have to testify against yourself, and only a fool would want to do that." As he walked me out he said he had no idea how much his handling of the case would cost; a lot would depend on whether or not it went before a jury. He requested, however, that for starters, "Leave a $10,000 retainer with my secretary."

For one, ethereal moment I'd considered telling Roth the truth, and then I thought better of it. The notion of doing the honorable, decent thing never occurred to me again. My unscrupulous mind, concerned with the overwhelming anxiety that would surely come about by exposing the truth about myself put a precipitous end to it.

As far as I was concerned, there was no longer any truth or even reality, for that matter. From what I'd read and seen on TV, no one ever told his lawyer the truth anyhow. Whoever heard of a murderer confessing to his lawyer? Hell, lawyers didn't even want to know the truth. That wasn't the object of the contest.

Even though I had purchased an ally, I was still anxious, since he had not, as yet, offered any encouragement or optimism other than the rather lame, "I'll do my best for you, try not to worry," cliché. Maybe, he wasn't buying my story.

A much more formidable task than fantasizing in front of a lawyer, and one that was making me even more anxious, was having to confront Hannah with the details of my plight. I had no choice but to tell her, inasmuch as my future was, to say the least, precarious. She, however, made it easy for me.

After emboldened by Darvon with a gulp of Maalox, I called and asked if I could come over. "There's something really important I need to discuss with you," I said.

"Don't bother," she countered, "I know exactly what's going on and am definitely not concerned. If you need someone to talk to or help you—which I doubt anyone can—get a lawyer. For God's sake, asshole, do something right for a change!"

The next time I saw Roth, he brought me up to date. "I just got off the phone with the Assistant U.S. Attorney, Artemis Bledsoe," he said. "He went over your case with me. Shortly after your hearing, the FDA turned what it had on you over to the Consumer Affairs Section of the Justice Department. They were sure it was enough to get a grand jury to indict. Their office, however, was so loaded down, they didn't get to it until three months ago. Since then, they've been corroborating the evidence the FDA investigators dug up from interviewing 30 of the 45 patients whose names they found on both the case study forms and on your office records. All of them denied having participated in any drug study, and they all said they would testify against you."

He then asked me if I knew who any of those patients were. I told him, "maybe 15 or 20, since they had personally called me."

"What did you tell them?"

"I said there had been some mix up in our research records, and that I wasn't sure how or why, but that Vern had somehow mistakenly used their names, that we were looking into the matter, and not to worry. I was sure it was an honest mistake."

After acknowledging my answer with a curt nod, he sat there staring blankly into space, both hands cupping his chin, elbows braced on the rosewood. After a while, he sighed deeply and murmured exasperatingly, "I know you told the FDA all your records regarding the clinical trials were destroyed, but go on and check your files again anyhow. At least get the records of the ones who called you. I need to see them."

I left, sure that Roth knew I was a shameless liar, that I was guilty, and that Vern was nothing but a scapegoat.

RABBI SCHACHNER

One morning in early spring, while Cavendish was making his weekly inspection of the toilets, I asked him if it would be possible for me to have a word with a rabbi. Cav soon followed through. He soon summoned Rabbi Aaron Schachner, a diminutive, balding saint who, *just like that*, helped me through my religious crisis.

The day was exploding with sun and the buds on the trees were starting to burst into pale-green leaves so I took Rabbi Schachner out to the gazebo, where he reached into his satchel and gave me precious gifts. Along with a pocket-sized prayer book, he handed me a brown bag that held a picnic: a kosher corned beef sandwich and a can of Dr. Brown's cream soda: still cold. My heart filled with love.

We chatted for a few minutes about family, careers, and the hostages in Iran as I munched and gulped, and then sitting on the towel I had brought for him, he listened pensively with pursed lips and an occasional nod as I sketched the particulars of my life and of my recent flirtation with evangelical Christianity. And then, I listened.

"Jim," he smiled empathetically, "even if you stopped believing or even hate our God because you blame Him for your troubles, you're still a Jew. You can't stop being a Jew. Even if you become a danger to yourself or, for that matter, the whole world, you're still a Jew. You will always belong.

"It doesn't really matter what religion you choose to practice. Any religion, as long as it explains life and death—or tries to—and teaches its members how to live a virtuous life, is doing what it's supposed to do. Frankly, Jim, they all do. Churches, temples, and mosques have nothing to do with the spirituality of a person. It's only the use of the wisdom and the judgment you've been given to cope with the trials of your existence, and to make the world a better place that count. There's no such thing as a superior religion."

"But, Rabbi, I though Judaism was. Aren't we supposed to be the chosen ones?"

"Oh-h-h, my God," he burst out laughing, "that's gotta be the *heder* in you coming out. The epithet, "chosen," by no means implies some exclusive possession of God's love or that other people are inferior. It only means that God has the exclusive rights to our service and obedience. We're not masters: we're servants! During our lives on *this* planet, He wants us to help fulfill His plan—the formation of a universal brotherhood. As opposed to Christianity, there is no promise of a reward after death for good behavior. Judaism is a religion of *this* world. It's objective, or as we say in the business, desideratum, is to 'do unto others as you would have them do unto you.'

"Listen, Jim, I've gotta run. I have a lecture to give over at the University of Richmond, and I mustn't be late. How 'bout let's continue this next week, say over another corned beef?"

VERNON

One evening, less than two weeks before the grand jury was to convene, I received a collect call from Vern. He said he was calling from "LA County," where a few days before, he'd had some sort of surgery on his leg. When he awoke from the anesthetic, there were two visitors sitting at his bedside, an FDA agent and a federal marshal. Before he had a chance to blink, they had served him with a subpoena to appear before the same grand jury I had been cordially invited to.

He didn't know what to do. He was alone, had no money, and had been living for several months out of a suitcase in various missions.

His mind was muddled, and at times he was crying, pressing me to do something. I knew he must be suffering the anguish of withdrawal, had undergone surgery simply to get narcotics, and his doctors, by now, were probably ignoring his pleas. He was unhinged, going around in circles, rattled and volatile. He was asking me for help, either that or telling me I was the cause of his having hit rock bottom, and I better damn well take care of him or else! The "or else" being, he would spill his guts out to the FDA. It was frightening, and I knew I was going to have to do something.

I suspected the government had probably done a background check on him, and discovered he had neither the intelligence, the training, nor the motive to fabricate these sophisticated, clinical investigations. They had to be chomping at the bit to get me, having figured out I had, somehow, conned Vern into taking much of the blame. I envisioned them granting him immunity in order to use him as a material witness against me. But, I assumed, *if he wasn't around, they could never prove what role I played. And if he wasn't around, what was to stop me from alleging he did it all?* With Vern out of the way, there was a chance I could walk away from this mess, scot-free! I had to get him out of Smog City, and fast.

I told him to stay by the phone. I'd call him back in an hour. I hung up, called United, drove down to National, paid cash for a ticket on the red-eye, and then called him back from a pay phone in the airport. Sure enough: he answered.

☙

It had taken Bledsoe several days to present the evidence and his witnesses, but it had taken only a few minutes for all 23 jurists to agree there was more than enough probable cause to indict both Vern and me on 19 felony charges: five counts of mail fraud, two counts of wire fraud, and 12 counts of writing fraudulent and false documents; all being felonious violations of Title 18 of the United States Code, Sections 1341, 1343, and 1001, and each punishable by a fine of up to $10,000 and/or imprisonment up to five years. If we got the "max," I quickly calculated, it would cost us each $190,000 and 95 years in prison.

When Roth phoned to break the news, he mentioned that the government's legal team was quite disturbed over the fact, that after catching up with Vern, he had somehow slipped through their fingers. "They had granted him full immunity and were all set to take him into custody and bring him back here to testify against you at the grand jury. Without his testimony, they can't establish the exact extent of your involvement which they contend approaches 100 percent! But even without it, they're confident they have enough on you to take the case to a jury: specifically the 30 witnesses they have who will swear you not only improvised their taking part in clinical investigations, but that you or someone forged their signatures. And, Bledsoe tells me, if he can convince the judge to allow it in, he's certain he'll be able to convince a jury, or at least instill doubt in their minds, as to your culpability regarding the break-ins at your office. The upshot is, they're pretty sure they have enough on you to put you behind bars.

"And, if they do find Vern, and he testifies for the government, it'll be an open and shut case. You'd probably end up with a stiff fine and at least 20 years.

"But, since a trial would be lengthy and costly, not only to the government, but to you as well, they've offered a plea bargain. Because of the amount of time, effort, and money they've already spent on this case, however, they are insisting on some jail time."

The Assistant District Attorney had conceded to drop all the charges but for a single count of making false statements to the government: a felony that mandated a sentence of up to five years in prison and a fine of up to $10,000. Roth felt the offer quite reasonable seeing as I now had no one to give credence to my lies.

RABBI SCHACHNER

The following week he came back as promised, bearing another corned beef sandwich gift. There was a light spring rain outside this time, so we had to sit at a card table in the visitors' room.

"Jim, you can't define God, nor can you visualize Him as a thing. He is not an object, or a man, and He doesn't live in some celestial space. He is a spiritual force, and He is here. He's always here. It's only us who are far away: oblivious. To find God, you must make yourself conscious of Him, and you must make yourself available to Him."

"You mean pray?"

"No, no, no. You can't have a true encounter with God simply by expressing your hopes and dreams to Him or by glorifying Him. To have a genuine relationship with God, you must truly meet with Him. The essence of our religion lies in having such rendezvous during which every aspect of one's life: every experience, every adversity, and every sorrow is scrutinized. Working together in such a manner with God helps you face and deal with life's challenges, but you have to, first, let Him inside you, for He only lives in those who let Him in."

"How, Rabbi?" I knew it couldn't be *just like that*.

"Like I said, He's here, and He wants to enter your world, mainly through the relationships you develop with people. But they must be honest, open, and shared: without pretense and without façades. In other words, being there . . . for someone . . . not for *your* sake but for *theirs*, and certainly not to exploit them as if they were things. Such relationships would be very conducive to your healing process, Jim, and they don't require drugs or a psychiatrist, just someone to talk to who cares. But you don't always need to say anything. In fact, the most emotional moments of life occur without a single word being spoken. Think about it. It's during such moments that one is having a true dialogue with God.

"By relating to others, Jim, you will gain control of your life. You will feel safe, and you will have faith in yourself, let alone the world. Faith will take the place of power: the double-dealing, bogus power that caused you to be manipulative and fraudulent. It will allow you to interact with people honestly, and to work together to solve the problems of life.

"The realization, Jim, of your potential as a human being demands such relationships. Finding yourself and relating to others will prove to be the most rewarding route to redemption.

"And incidentally, beautiful moments with music, poetry, art, and especially nature also offer occasions to meet God. Such aesthetic endeavors "say" something and, thus, there is dialogue. Just look around you. Don't tell me, He's not here."

Vern had been just a thing to me. He was a simple, innocent, crippled kid—a victim of poverty, polio . . . and me. Oh, God.

DENOUEMENT

found Vern on the floor in a shoddy room of the motel I had taken him to near the West Virginia border. He was half-way under the bed curled up like a fetus—naked—reeking of stale sweat, vomit, and cheap wine. For a moment I feared he was dead—perhaps even wishing he was—but he was warm and had a pulse. His skin had a saffron cast to it, and his belly was bloated. I soaked a towel in cold water and cowled his face with the dripping wetness. Five minutes later, he flung it off, and asked me where the hell I'd been for the past five days. I told him I was sorry, but that I'd been sick.

I sobered him up a bit with an ice-cold shower which he deeply resented. Leaving him in a bed that hadn't been made up in days, I went out and got him some buttered toast and a Coke which he promptly ate, and just as promptly puked up. After letting him sleep for an hour, I shook him awake, and guided his hand as I got him to copy and sign the self-damning confession I had written regarding his participation in the clinical trials.

Dear Sir,

When I was in LA, the FDA told me Dr. Scheiner faked the research he did for drug companies.

That is not true. The only thing he ever did was sign as the witness on the informed consent papers I would bring to him. Everything else was filled out by me.

I am writing this letter as I am too sick to testify for him, in person.

He had absolutely no idea what he had copied and signed.

Relieved and anxious to get away from that appalling scene, I threw some cash on the bedside table, restocked it with a hundred-capsule bottle of Pheraphen and my last three bottles of vintage red. I said I'd be back in two or three days, but he was snoring as I spoke. On my way out, I set the lock on the door, softly closed it, checked to be sure the "Do Not Disturb" sign was still there, and went to the manager's office to pay the clerk for five more days.

I got back home around seven, and drove straight to the lawyer's office, hoping to find him eclipsed behind his roll-top. He was. I apologized for the lateness of my visit, but explained that, "I had just gotten the mail, and found this note in the mailbox. I think it's important. There was no envelope." I could see, from the dubious half-smile on his face as he mouthed the words written in Vern's childish scrawl on the crumpled sheet of lined notebook paper that he thought something devious was going on, but he posed no questions and dismissed me by pithily saying he would show it to Bledsoe first thing in the morning.

Four days later Roth's secretary called to say he wanted to see me—urgently. Something was terribly wrong.

Roth looked at me with anger and disgust. Then, in a muted voice, he broke the news: "They found your friend . . . yesterday . . . just in time to save his life." He paused. "You are in deep shit."

He went on to say that Vern had been found unconscious and near death by one of the motel maids. He was bleeding from both his stomach and his pancreas, the morbid consequence of a deadly alliance of codeine, alcohol, and adversity. After emergency surgery, it was touch and go, made more so by the remorseless reality of withdrawal. But he survived to tell his story to his mother who, in turn, told the FBI.

Bledsoe was furious and appalled at my behavior, but regardless of what I had done to Vern, to him the worst crime of all was obstructing justice which he considered "a personal affront to the United States, and, on that account, unforgivable." If charged, Roth pointed out, it would be a crime he would have extreme difficulty defending simply because, like everything else I had done, there were no discernable, mitigating circumstances. "There can never be an excuse," he ranted, "for obstructing justice, Doctor. NEVER! But," he spit, "I'll do my best for you, as long as you realize the prognosis here is pretty grim, to say the least. Dammit, Doctor, that son-of-a-bitch almost died!"

The plea bargain had, of course, been withdrawn, and as to whether or not the "United States" would go on to charge me with obstruction, along with kidnapping, attempted manslaughter, distribution of narcotics, perjury, and God knows what else, was in a state of suspense. The Violations of Title 18 U.S.C., Section 1001 now seemed rather lame, and not worth mentioning.

It was bad enough listening to Roth delineate and dissect my cavalier crimes, but what hurt most was his unconcealed disappointment in my not having been honest with him. He was clearly pained that I hadn't trusted him or had faith in him. Still standing over me, he shook his head in regret.

The war was over. I had lost.

Strangely enough, I wasn't in a panic. Instead, I felt a sense of relief at being caught. I would be found guilty and go to prison, where I belonged.

Bledsoe now demanded I plead guilty to five of the 19 felony counts, but Roth somehow managed to get him down to three. I had no choice but to accept the offer. Artemis Bledsoe was indeed fair. And so, as the spire of the United States District Court for the Eastern District of Virginia on Washington Street in Old Town Alexandria was becoming mantled with snow, I pled guilty to the three counts.

Immediately, upon receiving the news of my sentencing, the Virginia State Board of Medicine revoked my license to practice medicine and surgery in their state.

My life as a Janus doctor was over.

APOLOGIA

April 14, 1981

Dear Vern,

I hope you haven't tossed out this letter, having seen my name on the envelope. Anyhow, if you have decided to read it, I'm very grateful. It's taken me a long time to get up the courage to write you this apology and to beg your forgiveness.

As you can see, I'm in the federal prison at Petersburg. It's in Southern Virginia near the North Carolina border. Yes, I know exactly what you're thinking. *I hope that bastard rots there.* I don't blame you at all. I deserve to be here.

I was sentenced to seven years in prison, but I got lucky, the judge suspended all but one year. After I get out, though, I'll be on probation for three years. I also lost my medical license, which I doubt I'll ever get back. I also lost Hannah and the kids. She hasn't asked for a divorce yet, but I'm sure it's coming.

Since being here and getting clean, I've tried to understand why I took advantage of our friendship and hurt you like I did. It was a horrible thing to do to someone who was always there for me. I now know that, besides being a drug addict, I was very, very sick. I was warped with corruption, selfishness, and greed. I was a real bastard, but I don't have to tell you that!

For whatever it means, I'll always regret the terrible wrongs I did to you, and, believe me, I know that neither my being sorry nor any amount of tears can ever make up for what I did. I wish I could heal your hurt, and I pray you'll be able to find it in your heart to forgive me, but if you can't, I'll understand. But I'll never stop praying that, someday, you will.

I hope you will at least accept as an apology the dreadful consequences on my life that resulted from my having betrayed your trust.

I pray you and your family are well, and may God bless you.

Jim

My letter to Vern was returned to me marked "NOT ACCEPTED BY ADDRESSEE."

PEACE

was lost in ambiguous thoughts as I blindly made my way up the serpentine path to the jogging track. About half-way up, I unconsciously stepped aside into the shrub to let someone, smelling of coconut pomade, by. But, instead, he halted and put a hand on my shoulder. I looked up, quizzically, when the tall mullato dressed Muslim-style in kaftan and kufi and leaning on a cane whispered, "I've been looking for you, Dr. Scheiner. Word is you're going home."

"Yes, that's right," I quavered, "tomorrow."

Antoine and I stood for a moment silently taking stock of each other until the warm smile sketching itself on his face unbolted my body and melted away my fear. He then reached for my hand and held it as he spoke. "I want you to know I'm thankful you were able to save my leg. Yes, Allahu akbar."

EPILOGUE

For most, prison is a boarding school for the study of crime. It is also an institution of higher learning for the vanguards of the most radical and desperate supremacy networks in America—black and white. *This* is their breeding and training grounds where crash courses in hate, taught by faculties of fanatical gurus, are extremely popular with the most enthusiastic and sincere of student bodies.

For some, however, prison is a sanitarium—a sanctuary—where even the most savage of miscreants have been known to experience a transcendent renascence, during which they are somehow freed from souls warped with malignant hostility and rancor. These, of course, are the blessed. I was one.

❧

Compared to the restless decay that is the Anacostia section of D.C., Petersburg was a paradise. The halfway house, claiming to be a place where felons are assisted in readjusting to society, was, in reality, nothing more than a temporary shelter run by a skeletal staff of self-important despots who couldn't have cared less about their responsibilities, let alone their "guests."

Over the years, the house, a derelict Georgian Revival that should have been condemned years ago, had been battered both inside and outside by the ordained petulance of its guests. Now barely livable, its rooms—whose walls were replete with crudely printed,

what-can-and-what-you-can't-do bulletins that only partially concealed the graffiti—walled in but a few, shoddy necessities. It was
situated right on the main drag, a "hardened artery" that existed primarily for the night. During the sun, it remained hushed and untrou-
bled, but once the stealthy shadows and the darkness settled in, it
burst forth with an inconceivable assortment of flakes, freaks, fantasies, and fluorescence, all charged with pretentious ribaldry.

This profane and boorish ambiance, along with my current vocation—car washer—just wasn't my penchant. All of a sudden, I missed
my calling. *My God*, I thought, *what the hell have I done, and, now, what
the hell am I gonna do?*

I phoned my lawyer, and, although his last words to me had been,
"Doc, you've been the most agonizing schmuck of a client I have ever
had. Puhleez, don't ever call me again!" he said he would try his best
to help me.

Predictably, his efforts to have my medical license reinstated were
futile. It had been revoked, and the state board felt it much too soon
to consider rescinding the order. It was ironic as hell, for had they
known I was a Janus doctor, chances are I would still be at work . . .
or dead.

Manny did find me a job, however, in of all places, Bahrain. He
had at one time gone over there to represent Aramco in some sort of
oil deal with the Amir. While there, he developed an acute bout of
appendicitis and had undergone surgery at the International Hospital,
a small private facility staffed by a cosmopolitan group of ex-pat doctors. As it turned out, orthopaedic surgeons—even iniquitous ones—
were in serious demand, there being only one on the entire island, and
he was with the competition at the government-controlled hospital
in al-Man☐ mah. Manny bluntly explained my circumstances to the
owner of the hospital who wasn't listening. He was only interested
in knowing when I could start, and if I would accept a tax-free salary
of $80,000 the first year. Trying hard not to laugh, he promised him

he would do his best to persuade me to take the job. It took just two more calls to get me over there: one to the Justice Department to have my passport returned, and one to the probation department to OK travel overseas.

When I started to thank him, he snarled, "Like I told you once before, the only thanks I want is to never see or hear from you again! Now give Esther a check for $5,000, and get the fuck out of here!" God, I felt bad. I knew he was serious. But more than that, I had no doubt I deserved his testy sentiments.

Less than a week, however, before I was due to wing over to the Persian Gulf, I thought my luck had run out. I was crouched down on my knees, fanatically buffing the hubcap on the right-rear tire of a slick, two-toned-blue Trans-Am when, as I started to stand up to admire its resplendent sparkle, something violently imploded deep within my left knee with a crack as sudden and as loud as a gunshot. It was so loud that some of my colleagues heard it even over the riotous fanfare of the slip-slopping, slam-bang sounds of the drive-through washer. The excruciating pain brought me back down on the slippery, soapy asphalt where I watched my knee puff up to at least the size of a bowling ball.

An ambulance took me to the Howard University Hospital ER where an orthopaedic resident drained at least a kegful of bloody-yellow gore out of it. After a CT scan revealed a huge tear of one of the cartilages, he admitted me to "ortho," and the following morning had me up in the OR where, at the largesse of the federal government, he performed arthroscopic surgery. I was discharged that evening and have never had a problem with that knee ever since. Hey, who was it said, "Black doctors are a joke?"

In Bahrain, treating appreciative Arabs and ex-pats, I, at long last, took pleasure in my profession. During the entire time I worked there, I never heard of or saw a Janus doctor. Harsh, absolute, and "persuasive" laws thwarted that sort of thing. I was also gratified to note the absence of malpractice suits, but human nature being what it is, professional jealousy and an obsession with luxury was just as ubiquitous and brazen.

I stayed on that scorched, petroleum-laden island until one blistering night, late, after leaving the brogue of a young, Irish songbird and more than a few empty bottles of San Miguel in the cabaret over at the Gulf Hotel, my phone rang.

I flinched at the quavering, "Dad?"

"Erich! Is that you?"

"Yeah."

"Something wrong?"

"No . . . no."

"Are your sure? Mom OK?"

"Yeah. Really! I was just calling to see if you could come home. I'll be graduating in three weeks, and I . . . I'd," he sobbed, "really like for you to be there. Can you?"

"Of course," I sighed tearfully, "I'll come."

"Thanks, Dad."

"Does Mom know you're calling me?"

"Uh-huh."

"What'd she say?"

"Actually, she asked me to call you."

"She did?!"

"Yeah. She told me to tell you, it was time for you to come home."

"Really?" I queried with a lightheaded grin.

"Oh, shit! Not you again."

"I'm sorry to bother you, Manny, but I'm back with Hannah, and was hoping you might see about getting my license back."

Even though armed with a stack of letters of thanks and recommendations from my colleagues in Bahrain as well as a couple of sheiks, the state of Virginia sent their regrets. Manny, however, was able to coax Texas into reinstating the license I had let lapse after completing my residency.

⚭

There weren't many places open, however, to a Janus doctor doing his best to prevail over a fractured career. Those that were were decaying rural towns where the oil used to gush and whose hospitals—anachronistic relics—were kept full by greedy quacks exploiting the system and their patients for all they could get. I wrestled with that contemptible mental climate for a few years, but when I sensed I realized I was at the brink of reopening an old wound, I had the good sense to quit.

It took a while, but Hannah and I succeeded in making a new beginning, full of promise. But just when the sun was shining, she began to complain of a gagging sensation while eating. Thinking it was from ill-fitting dentures, she consulted her dentist, but although he, an orthodontist, and an oral surgeon tried their best, it worsened, as did her disinterest in food. Within weeks, her shapely figure wasted away, her thick shag became wispy, and her eyes dulled. She finally consulted her family doctor. After a perfunctory exam, he told her she was depressed, and gave her some samples of Valium, none of which she took. Seeing as there was no pain, she decided to try and forget about it, perhaps fearing and in denial of the worst.

Three months after Hannah's elusive affliction began, the shampoo girl over at Josette's beauty salon thought her eyes looked "yellowish." By then, it was too late: the cancerous growth in her pancreas had become an egregious horror.

She slipped away three months later, but, during that ephemeral moment, together with a warm-hearted hospice team, I made certain she was kept comfortable and infused, along with her drips, with an eternity of love.

I only wish she had lived long enough to know that all four of her sons, unlike me, became doctors for all the right reasons.

AFTERWORD

"In the more than a century since Pasteur's time, medical science has raced ahead with astonishing speed to close in on some of the fundamental mysteries of life. And yet, we are no closer today than we ever were to resolving the problem of troubled physicians who are a danger to the well-being or even the lives of their patients."

Alan Bonsteel, M.D.

THE DISEASE

The AMA defines physician impairment as "the inability to practice medicine adequately by reason of physical or mental illness including alcoholism or drug dependence." The definition implies that the impaired judgment stemming from such diseases precludes the physician from determining whether or not he or she is competent to practice. Substance abuse accounts for the preponderance of such physicians.[1]

There are two, quintessential, occupational hazards of being a physician. The first—which is no secret, and owes its existence to a constant exercise of authority and self-love—is an outrageous, at times, farcical sense of omnipotence. The second is a progressive disease that has been allowed to reach epidemic dimensions, and owing to an irrational dilatoriness in its diagnosis and treatment invariably decays into either an appalling disability or death. The disease—chemical addiction.

The vulnerability of practicing physicians to this curse becomes apparent when one discovers that more or less 15 percent of them[2]— from that tender-hearted, white-haired general practitioner to that arrogant, urbane, young surgeon, but, uniquely, the behind-the-curtain anesthesiologist—are, at any one time, addicted to alcohol, to other drugs, or to both. As a consequence of their spurious invincibility, many of those so afflicted find it impossible to accept the fact that the abuse of drugs leads to addiction, and the fact that addiction, in turn, destroys the individualism they proclaim to be the very essence of their calling.

At the present time, of the roughly 872,000 physicians practicing in the United States, more or less 130,800 of them are chemically impaired: Janus doctors who, as a rule, do not stop seeing patients while stoned or sloshed. Physicians routinely see at least 60 patients per week. In starkest terms, this means that the Janus doctors, during a 48-week work year treat some 376,740,000 unsuspecting, innocent men, women, and children, if for no other reason than to maintain their gilt-edged lifestyles.

Although physicians have the same risk of alcoholism (± 10 percent) as the general public, they are, ironically, remarkably susceptible to drug addiction—up to seven times more—and which is usually accompanied by serious psychiatric afflictions.[3]

୧∼୨

Chemical addiction is the leading cause of physician impairment, and has been for at least the last half century. The true prevalence of drug dependency is probably much more than the estimated 15 percent inasmuch as most addicted physicians deny the fact. They conceal their craving, and, as a result of denial and self-deception in addition to the obstinate conspiracy of silence of their colleagues, are never discovered or treated. And unless, because of it, some catastrophic event intrudes—either to themselves or to their patients—they will take their depravity to their graves. The full extent of the problem is also deprecated seeing as how medical licensing and regulatory boards often under-report disciplinary actions, mortality statistics, and treatment records of impaired physicians.

Furthermore, these estimates do not include the thousands who practice while under treatment with psychoactive drugs prescribed by other doctors or by themselves, nor those who, while yet not dependent on drugs, take them to stay awake, get high, or to fool themselves into thinking such poisons improve their performance. For those responsible for human life, such insouciant use has real consequences as potentially devastating as addiction since the physiological and psychological effects of mind-altering substances are so unpredictable and so profound that attempting to treat patients, let alone operate on them, even after consuming a single dose is derelict, reprehensible, and potentially catastrophic, and the jeopardy may persist for prolonged periods of time, inasmuch as the elimination of such drugs from the body can be quite slow. A single dose of Prozac, for example, remains in one's bloodstream for more than a week. These chemicals dull the mental processes associated with memory, judgment, comprehension, and thinking, have a disturbing effect on coordination and dexterity, and, by inhibiting anxiety and guilt, provoke a heightening of one's self-confidence. Judgment and common sense may become so impaired that a physician becomes incapable or unwilling to objectively evaluate his or her capabilities, often believing they can do more than they could sober.

Early on, when taking drugs in moderation, a doctor's life becomes a satisfying experience: no longer a bitch. Their bedside manner and façade of caring become conspicuously impassioned, even a bit tawdry, but nevertheless convincing, for *then* they are still in control. As a result, in no time at all, the practices of these apocryphal "Albert Schweitzers" crescendo, simply because their performances are eaten up, blown up, and bandied about, by their naïve patients.

It is when they start—usually sooner than later—to want more of the wonders inherent in their soulless medication, such as transport to some celestial paradise, that the elixir now takes control, and begins to sow the scorching seeds of sorrow, pain, and hopelessness.

Then the drug becomes a savage demon, possessing unconditionally and totally the body in which it dwells. It will denature it and degenerate it, and, before long, it will turn it into a Janus: a healer with two faces: one moral, sincere, careful, strong, sober, and helpful; the other, immoral, deceitful, careless, weak, intemperate, and neglectful. A healer who, by harming himself, will inevitably inflict harm on those he once swore an oath to help and comfort.

❧

Owing to the inevitability that physicians who maltreat themselves will maltreat their patients, anyone, no matter who, setting foot into a medical facility—be it a hospital, emergency room, clinic, doctor's office, nursing center, or surgicenter, no matter what—whether it be for treatment of a mole or a malignancy, ought to ask, "When or if I leave here, will I be better or will I be worse?"

There's a damn good chance you'll be worse: a victim, but hardly a martyr, of a medical mistake. You may be misdiagnosed. You may be poisoned by being given the wrong medicine or the wrong dose, and end up clamped to a dialysis machine. You may have the wrong breast, or the wrong leg removed. You may wake up touch-and-go in an intensive care unit, having had a sharp or even a dull, surgical instrument slash through your esophagus, your womb, or a major blood vessel. You might even leave this world, surreptitiously, in a plastic, body bag through the back door. Yes, there's a damn good chance you may very well regret having sought medical treatment.

A Harris Poll taken in 1997 disclosed that one out of every three persons had been victims of medical mistakes.[4] Two years later, the National Academy of Sciences, after probing into an endless maze of medical mistakes, made the fourth estate ever more obtrusive than it usually is with the revelation that three million, medical errors that bring about nearly 100,000 deaths occur in American hospitals every year. Seeing as 70 percent of them are preventable, it makes American "healers" perpetrators of the eighth leading cause of death—iatrogenesis: a phenomenon that kills more people than motor vehicle accidents, breast cancer, or AIDS do.[5] Dr. Barbara Starfield of the Johns Hopkins School of Hygiene and Public Health, however, believes such errors result in 225,000 deaths per year which would be the equivalent of a jumbo jet crashing, without survivors, every day of the year, and would make it the third leading cause of death following heart disease and cancer.[6] Regardless, these are only the gaffes that happen inside hospitals. The three million become relatively inconsequential when one considers the multitudes of sick and injured that frequent all the other facilities where doctors ply their trade.

The burning question is, of course, how many of these mistakes and deaths come about at the hands and melted minds of Janus doctors? No doubt, a considerable number. Optimal medical care cannot be delivered by those whose passion and pursuit are no longer patient care, but, rather, the procurement and misuse of drugs.

There are a few professions where human error can lead to cataclysm, and thus cannot, under any circumstance, be tolerated. Extreme control systems have been set up striving to prevent needless accidents and deaths from nuclear warheads negligently exploding, from ships running aground, from commercial jets crashing, or from trains colliding. It goes without saying that such systems, which are vigorously enforced, include the prevention and immediate detection of alcohol and drug use by the personnel involved.

The men and women in these professions understand and accept such surveillance, for they are well aware of the potential consequences of carrying out their tasks with drugs impacting on their thoughts and on their physical reactions. They know, when it comes to drugs and alcohol, there can be no *laissez faire*. Consequently, mistakes, accidents, and deaths in these professions are rare. For example, the likelihood of being killed in a domestic jet flight is estimated to be one in eight million. In their worlds, there is no having to contend with 100,000 preventable fatalities yearly.

Yet in medicine, those responsible for countless numbers of human lives every minute of every day, and whose moral precept is *primum non nocere* (above all, do no harm) remain virtually unchecked despite their policy-makers being well aware of a very ominous situation.

೨೦

Countless accounts of addicted doctors began appearing in the medical literature over fifty years ago. But it was not until 1972 that the AMA chose to look into the matter and disinter the problem, but other than a few perfunctory recommendations, no one really got too excited over it. Reports of the problem, however, continued coming in, like the 1986 one from Harvard[7] that laid bare the particulars of the ten percent of doctors in an undisclosed New England state that were using drugs on a daily basis, and of the 48 percent of the state's psychiatrists, 44 percent of the anesthesiologists, 23 percent of the surgeons, and 17 percent of the obstetricians-gynecologists who were treating themselves with psychoactive drugs that included such magic bullets as Heroin, Demerol, Morphine, and LSD. Nevertheless, the researchers had the audacity to proclaim one of the most thoughtless and irrational conclusions of all time when they wrote, ". . . the overall level of psychoactive drug use . . . should not be cause for great alarm," even though they suspected it was on the rise. I'm sure they'd be alarmed, though, if one of those dope-dabbling doctors was performing surgery on them.

In 1992, a report published in the Journal of the American Medical Association stated that 10.4 percent of all physicians drank alcohol on a daily basis,[8] and the next year, the Medical College of Wisconsin reported that one in six of the anesthesiologists who had trained there confessed to being a Janus doctor, yet not one ever had their license to practice suspended, or had any disciplinary action taken relative to substance abuse.[9] This would explain why a report from the Duke University Medical Center published in 2002 stated that the frequency of drug abuse among anesthesiologists had not significantly changed.[10] In fact, it was on the rise as evidenced by a report published in 1999 that stated as many as 18 percent of all doctors were abusing drugs or alcohol,[11] or as Dr. Robert Coombs believed, it was crescendoing, and the true incidence was more like 20 percent.[12]

Seemingly indifferent to the reports that have been piling up regarding a profession pregnant with potential criminals, the AMA remains blatantly jaundiced. They insist substance abuse by physicians is neither outstanding nor a cause for concern. In a rather cavalier fashion, they dispatch the problem as being inconsequential. That such is their conviction is evident by their declaration that, "nevertheless," they would continue to look after the needs of impaired physicians which, of course, implied concealing and sheltering them through its Physician Health Program. No mention was ever made, however, of looking after the safety of millions of patients.[13] It is nothing less than pathetic that a supposedly principled, scientific body, in order to preserve the reverence and homage its members believe is their due, must resort to deception.

And so it is that Janus doctors continue to thrive.

The testing of promising drugs in humans proceeds through three phases. Phase I consists of trying out the investigational drug on a small number of both healthy subjects and those with the target disease to determine what happens to the drug once it gets in the body from a metabolic and toxic point of view. If things look good after this small but important launch, Phase II studies are then initiated using a larger number of patients. This group is used to assess the efficacy of the drug, and to note the type and incidence of side effects. Should the drug show promise, Phase III studies drawing on a large-scale series of patients—anywhere from 500 to several thousand—are then set in motion to gather as much information as possible in order to evaluate the overall benefit/risk ratio which, if found convincing, is then submitted for approval by the FDA. The entire process may take as long as a decade to complete.

Before the FDA descended upon the pharmaceutical industry back in the '60s, clinical investigations were carried out in the ivory towers of academic medicine. Now, because of the sizable numbers of patients required to measure the safety and effectiveness of a drug, and to have them approved as quickly as possible, the industry makes use of the private sector. It has always been difficult, however, to recruit private practitioners: that is, honest ones. They neither have the time nor the inclination to test experimental drugs on their patients, not only because of the exacting standards for such investigations demanded by the FDA, but because of the anxiety of knowing that some of their patients would be taking placebos or would develop complications which could ignite legal action.

Unfortunately then, many of the doctors inclined to conduct clinical trials are the greedy, the needy, and the dregs which spells out why Phase III studies are tainted by a broad spectrum of malfeasance. In fact, a decade after I was convicted, more than 11 percent of the investigational trials audited by the FDA were found to have egregious instances of fraud that included gross fabrications of patient and lab results, enrollment of inappropriate subjects, and failure to obtain informed consent.[14] This prompted the FDA to encourage pharmaceutical firms to train and have monitors regularly visit trial sites in order to make certain investigators were not falsifying data. As a result, in 1994, the instances of egregious deficiencies dropped to five percent.[15]

Over the past few years, however, that trend seems to have reversed itself owing to a drastic metamorphosis that has taken place in the practice of medicine—managed care. To the bitter dismay of the vast majority of doctors, practice incomes have plunged.

Managed care has also put a crunch on the cost of drugs which has effectively suppressed the profits of their manufacturers. To remain competitive and to please their shareholders, pharmaceutical companies have been pressured into increasing the number of developmental drugs in their "pipelines." The rivalry has become cutthroat, and, as a result of the FDA having recently stepped up its approval process for NDAs, speed, more than ever, is of the essence. Clinical trials have become like NASCAR trials, using patients instead of cars. Unfortunately, pharmaceutical firms can't manufacture patients. They have to rely on doctors to enlist the armies of patients needed. And they're getting them simply by dispensing outrageous sums of money to the doctors performing their clinical trials, or by paying them just as much or more for recruiting patients to participate in trials being performed by a newly contrived, lucrative, medical specialty—clinical trialists. Phase III research has become an assembly line industry that bestows upon its operatives an overwhelming incentive to cheat.

Hundreds of thousands, perhaps millions, of patients have already been recruited for this thriving, multibillion-dollar business. Over the past ten years, the number of clinical trialists in the United States has tripled. And why not? Many are making over million dollars each year.

And so the drug firms are getting their guinea pigs, but, in doing so, they have bluntly intruded their own concerns into the ticklish relationship that exists between a patient and his doctor, and, sadly, the patients aren't even aware of it. Even worse, as a result of "drugola," a doctor's judgment, as often as not, becomes torn between passing up a quick profit or enrolling an innocent patient in an inappropriate, potentially injurious, even fatal study. Money, being the great corrupter of judgment, invariably wins by consciously or unconsciously goading doctors to minimize the dangers or maximize the benefits of the drug in order to persuade patients to pollute their bodies with something they really don't need. And so the patient, rather than being a sick or injured person, has now become an uncaged laboratory animal.

Some time ago, the executives of Merck & Company, during the clinical trials of their antihypertensive drug, Cozaar, became nervous upon learning their trialists were having trouble finding enough, qualified patients. At first, they had been offering $2,995 for each patient enrolled in the study. In an effort to stimulate their doctors to "deliver," they offered them a $500 bonus for each patient, and if they were able to enlist fourteen patients by a certain date, they were rewarded with an additional $2,000: a package deal worth over $50,000! Merck got their patients, but we'll never know how many of these patients were not qualified to be in the study, nor how many were actually harmed. It's intriguing to imagine how, if the patients just aren't there, incentive pay can, somehow, make them appear. This alchemistic phenomenon known as "massaging entry criteria," is prevalent throughout the pharmaceutical industry.[16]

As a consequence, the business of Phase III studies has been placed, more than ever, under a very dark, very suspicious cloud. There is no doubt, many of these trialists are corrupt charlatans: unqualified, inexperienced, and totally uninterested in anything other than their IRAs. And, yes, probably many are Janus doctors. But one thing is certain, the pharmaceutical firms know exactly what's going on, but in their jungle such things are often winked at.

THE ANTIDOTE

Roughly 90 percent of all drug offenders convicted in federal courts are sentenced to prison, accounting for 59 percent of the federal prison population. The state courts are a bit more lenient. Of those who defy their drug statutes and are busted, 72 percent end up in prison. There, they make up 21 percent of the inmate population.[17]

If 15 percent of doctors are impaired by chemicals, then every day 15 percent of doctors break the law. Yet the number of Janus doctors, according to a spokesperson for the National Association of State Controlled Substances Authorities (NASCSA), in either system is inconsequential, "probably not more than two dozen in the nation," It is, indeed, an uneven playing field.[18]

How is it that so many doctors, in so many communities, in so many medical facilities in the United States buy, steal, and use dangerous drugs with relative impunity? It was a Mansfield, Ohio, detective, Robert Mortimer, who disclosed the cold, hard truth when he said, "You can go out and bust the cokers and the dopers and the junkies and bring them to court, no problem. You move uptown and start messing with the doctors, though, and everybody backs off."[19] Although his statement was made back in 1985, it remains an inescapable fact to this day. Clearly and undeniably, doctors *are* above the law. When it comes to alcohol and drugs, they play by their own rules, and nearly all get away with it for far too long, which is usually after they make some distressingly deadly blunder. Even then, the impulse of those in charge is not to press for automatic punishment, but, rather, to cover it up as best they can.

The treatment of this disease in doctors is strikingly different from anyone else who acquires it. The medical profession considers chemical addiction a disease, but one with two disparate divisions: one that only seizes doctors, and is treated with TLC, concern, and confidentiality, and the other that seizes everyone else, but which is treated with condemnation, prosecution, and exile. The truth is, the divisions are nothing more than a specious dichotomy that smacks of prejudice and discrimination.

So, why isn't everyone damned by drugs treated the same? All other diseases are. If a doctor gets gonorrhea, *he* gets penicillin. If a hooker gets gonorrhea, *she* gets penicillin. Why are Janus doctors considered special, and when caught, treated with indulgence or concerned neglect? Why are the drug abusers in our glutted prisons not treated similarly? There is no justification for those guilty of abusing drugs, and who, by doing so, jeopardize their patients' lives, not to be punished like everyone else by the criminal justice system, and, for knowingly scorning their professional responsibilities and the trust of their patients, disciplined by the State Boards of Medicine, as well.

Putting an abrupt end to the impaired physician's privilege to practice medicine, exposing his or her criminal activities, and, perhaps, throwing him or her in the slammer would not only safeguard the public, but could very well act as a deterrent to those disposed on embarking on that voyage to hell. And the same goes for those who fail to inform on their colleagues who they know or suspect of using drugs. Both state and federal laws dictate that any licensed, health-care practitioner must report not only overt but possibly impaired physicians to the State Board of Medicine. Nevertheless, it remains almost unheard of for doctors to snitch on an impaired colleague. Instead, they close their eyes. They would much rather believe his or her curious, unconventional, or bizarre behavior is related to personality quirks, fatigue, or stress. The problem with that agenda is, Janus doctors are already choked with denial. Unable to recognize their affliction, they refrain from seeking help. Entry into treatment must, therefore, be instigated by others, but if all the others are in denial, what chance have they?

That doctors are above the law is attributable, not only to this "conspiracy of silence," but to the charitable and dilatory behavior of the State Boards of Medicine, as well. Summoned before these self-regulatory cliques, a Janus doctor can anticipate, at most, a sympathetic rebuke or a recommendation to seek treatment, for what is, undeniably, flagrant criminal activity. The majority of Janus doctors are never punished or prohibited—even temporarily—from practicing medicine, and their identities, seldom released to the public. Should the rare instance occur where an impaired physician is arrested and convicted, even then the Board will refuse to act until the conviction is upheld on appeal, no matter how far it is taken nor how long it takes. Their position being, if they took away a doctor's license, and the conviction was overturned, the doctor would have lost his license for nothing. As a result, convicted Janus doctors are often allowed to remain in practice and unpunished for years.

Although mandated by law to protect the public, medical boards seem more concerned with concealing Janus doctors from public exposure than with the safety of patients, and despite all having established programs to deal with Janus doctors there has been no attrition in its pervasiveness. These purported Impaired Physician Programs contain experts in the treatment of addictive disorders who have drawn up educational programs to instruct doctors on how to identify their addicted colleagues, and the appropriate techniques for intervention. They have, however, been anything but successful.

One of the most vocal critics of these programs, and justifiably so, is the Public Citizen's Health Research Group, a nonprofit consumer organization that monitors the activities of State Medical Boards. This organization probed into the records of disciplinary actions against all American doctors from 1987 until 1996. Of 2,322 disciplinary actions for substance abuse, only 538 doctors (41 percent) were ordered to stop seeing patients, many only temporarily. The rest were allowed to continue practicing. The brutal fact they were Janus doctors was concealed from their patients. And, unbelievably, less than 10 percent were ordered to obtain treatment, of which half hurriedly dropped out. Tragically, even now, these statistics remain essentially unchanged. In fact, in 2011, the "Research Group" reported that most state medical boards were still under-disciplining physicians, and were doing so less than they had in 1996. The members of the group were particularly alarmed over the fact that many of the Janus doctors were allowed to return to practice even after several attempts at rehabilitation had failed, or before they had fully recovered—if there is such a thing. And many, even after repeated acts of incompetence or negligence, were never disciplined. The fact remains, an army of Janus doctors exists "out there," maiming, defrauding, assaulting and murdering patients simply because no one wants to disclose their "dirty little secrets"! [20]

The State Boards of Medicine, in their silence, tolerance, and indecisiveness are putting the careers of such physicians above the safety of the public. In doing so, they are deliberately violating both the Medical Practice Act and the Controlled Substances Act. They justify their injurious actions by pointing out that addiction is a disease, and, as such, requires treatment, not disciplinary measures. But is that enough justification to allow an addicted physician who is in withdrawal, or being treated, or who relapses, to look after trusting, innocent patients?

The medical profession, in order to preserve, and perhaps even resuscitate the trust of society, must make a concerted effort to track down and prevent physicians who jeopardize themselves and, more importantly, their patients by the personal use of illicit drugs and alcohol. They must offer the assurance and security to the public that its members will do no harm, and if it can't, or won't, then the public has no choice, but to create the necessary strategies to do so.

Throughout the past few decades, remarkable breakthroughs and innovations concerning the causes of diseases, their diagnoses and their treatment have been made, yet the abuse of chemicals remains, not only the nation's number one health problem, but the medical profession's, as well. This crisis demands closure.

⁂

Self-regulation is the hallmark of a profession. It is an exceptional concession given in return for exceptional endeavors. It is a privilege the medical establishment has, when dealing with its impaired, been anything but compliant, if not promiscuous. This reluctance to act is clearly because doctors practice their art in an unwavering state of uncertainty in an environment conducive to perpetrating mistakes. It is a backdrop of frustration brought on by swarms of patients with unrealistic expectations. It is this awkward uneasiness that has forged a compelling and loyal sense of collective sympathy and shared vulnerability amongst the profession. And so, it is no wonder they all tend to forgive and forget.

The solution to the problem seems straightforward: shift the profession from one that prompts its membership to obfuscate its flaws to one that seeks help by bringing them out into the open. But doing so is no easy affair, for even if the crucial obstacle to treatment—denial—is surmounted, the guilt and shame of their bitter pill will, perhaps even more so, restrain them from reaching out.

Purging the Janus doctors out of the profession demands a comprehensive, sweeping, national agenda. This agenda must begin early on in medical school with putting an end to unwarranted sources of stress, with a concerted psychological screening of applicants, and by

assisting students in developing coping skills to deal with the anticipated unexpected.

Students and physicians at all levels of training must also receive
an eclectic education as to the causes, characteristics, and prevention
of drug and alcohol abuse so as to be able to identify the problem and
intervene as early as possible. This would assure better therapeutic
results, and help dispel the delusion that physicians are immune from
such lunacy.

Such conventional measures, along with tight drug controls are,
of course, important and necessary, but, by now, they have all been set
in motion and have all proved to be in vain. What is needed, because
we are concerned with human lives, is a bold, zero-tolerance strategy
which means the case for mandatory drug screening becomes relevant.

At the present time, the AMA—ever-protective of its members—
does not endorse drug testing of physicians. They claim it only pro-
vides limited information, and seriously intrudes on personal privacy.
Such objections are, strictly speaking, excuses, and hardly convincing
when you're trying to de-escalate three million mistakes and up to
225,000 needless deaths year in and year out. When done properly
and frequently on everyone, employing forensically defensible, chain-
of-custody documentation, it would have a consummate impact on
the problem of Janus doctors. After identifying a substance-abusing
doctor, he or she would then be referred for appropriate treatment,
and, at the same time, the State Board of Medicine and the appropriate drug enforcement agency alerted.

There are few activities in our society more personal or private
than the passing of urine. Watching someone urinate is undeniably
an intrusion, an invasion, and an imposition. But what is more important: a patient's life or a brief moment of embarrassment? Witnessed
collection is imperative in order to avoid a sham specimen. Unless
observed closely, Janus doctors, being very crafty, can easily substitute
their specimens with apple juice or someone else's urine, or "doctor"

them with a whole slew of substances such as salt, vinegar, ammonia, soap, or Clorox that make accurate, chemical analysis impossible. Desperate addicts have even been known to instill someone else's urine into their own bladders by using a catheter, and, some have even used artificial penises that contain a reservoir for holding someone else's specimen. Eclipsing these techniques, however, is the use of artificial urine, available from Byrd Laboratories down in Austin, Texas who, along with your purchase, includes a pamphlet entitled, Conquering the Urine Tests!

Random drug testing is an effective system by which those who take drugs can be identified and, hopefully, dealt with before harm is done. The public needs such responsible assurance from the medical profession: a profession which, over the past few decades has made imposing advances in finding the causes of diseases, their diagnoses and their treatment, yet the use and abuse of drugs and alcohol remain, not only the nation's foremost health problem, but the medical profession's, as well. Despite everything, it *is* open to solution.

Endnotes

1. AMA Council on Mental Health: The sick physician: impairment by psychiatric disorders, including alcoholism and drug dependence. JAMA 1973; 223: 684-687.
2. Bohigian, G.M., Croughan, J.L., Sanders K. Substance abuse and dependence in physicians: an overview of the effects of alcohol and drug abuse. Missouri Med 1994; 91: 233-238; Farley, W.J., Talbott, G.D. Anesthesiology and addiction. Anesth Analg 1983; 62: 465-6; Flaherty, J.A., Richman, J.A. Substance use and addiction among medical students, residents, and physicians. Psychiatr Clin North Am 1993; 16: 189-197; Moore, R.D., Mead, L., Pearson, T.A. Youthful precursors of alcohol abuse in physicians. A J Med 1990; 88: 332-336; Centrella, M. Physician addiction and impairment—current thinking: a review. J Add Dis 1994; 13: 91-104; Spiegelman, W.G., Saunders, L., Mazze, R.I. Addiction and anesthesiology. Anes 1984; 60: 335-341; Setness, P.A. A sobering look at our profession. Post Grad Med 1995; 98: 15-27; and Keith, J.F. Into the next century: A strategic plan for the North Carolina physicians' health program. NCMJ 1996; 57: 243-245. Hughes, P.H., Brandenburg, N., Baldwin, D.C., et al. Prevalence of substance use among US physicians. JAMA 1992; 267: 2333-2339.
3. Spiegelman, W.G., Saunders, L., Mazze, R.I. Addiction and anesthesiology. Anesthesiology 1984: 60: 335-341.

4. Levy, D. Medical mistakes happen to many, AMA poll finds. USA Today. 1997; Oct. 10-12.

5. Lemonick, M.D. Doctor's deadly mistakes. Time. 1999; Dec 13: 74-76.

6. Starfield, B. Is US health really the best in the world? JAMA 2000; 284: 483-485.

7. McAuliffe, W.E., Rohman, M., Santangelo, D.A., et al. Psychoactive drug use among practicing physicians and medical students. NEJM 1986; 315: 805-10.

8. Hughes, P.H., Brandenburg, N., Baldwin, D., et al. Prevalence of substance abuse among US physicians. JAMA 1992; 267: 2333-2339.

9. Lutsky, I., Hopwwod, M., Abram, S.E. et al. Psychoactive substance use among anesthesiologists: a 30-year retrospective study. Can J. Anaesth 1993; 40: 915-21.

10. Booth, J.V., Grossman, D., Moore, J., et al. Substance abuse among physicians: a survey of academic anesthesiology programs. Anesth analg 2002; 95: 1024-1030.

11. Rice, B. Impaired physicians: giving rehab programs a new look. Medical Economics 1999; 76: 173-178.

12. Coombs, R.H. Drug-impaired Professionals, Cambridge, Massachusetts: Harvard University Press; 1997.

13. AMA Council on Mental Health. Report on the Council on Scientific Affairs: Substance Abuse Among Physicians. Chicago: American Medical Association; 1994.

14. Shapiro, M.F., Charrow, R.P. The role of data audits in detecting scientific misconduct: Results of the FDA program. JAMA 1989; 261: 2505-2511.

15. Cohen, J. Clinical trial monitoring: hit or miss? Science 1994; 264: 1534-1538.

16. Eichenwald, K., Kolata, G. Drug trials hide conflicts for doctors. The New York Times. 1999; May 16.

17. Maguire, K., Pastore, A.L., eds. Sourcebook of Criminal Justice Statistics, 2002. U.S. Department of Justice, Bureau of Justice Statistics. Washington D.C.: USGPO, 2003.

18. Personal communication.

19. Webb, G. Board leaves police disgusted, angry. The Plain Dealer. Cleveland. 985; April 9: 11-a.

20. Wolfe, S., 20,125 Questionable Doctors Disciplined by State and Federal Governments. Washington D.C.: Public Citizen Health Research Group: 2000.